"In *Hello Baby, Goodbye Intrusive Thoughts*, Jenny Yip decon[structs mater]nal anxiety and provides practical tools for stopping the [spiral]. The applications and sound advice of this book stretch fr[om treat]ing obsessive-compulsive disorder (OCD) to good advice f[or all moms. *Hello*] *Baby, Goodbye Intrusive Thoughts* is an important resource for all the many moms out there who deserve reprieve from the traps of anxiety, guilt, and exhaustion."

> —**Mali Heled Kinberg, PhD**, professor at the UCLA School of Theater,
> Film and Television; and the Anderson School of Management

"Jenny Yip expertly dives deep into the struggles generated by intrusive thoughts and postpartum anxiety, shedding light on a topic often shrouded in silence. She bravely shares her own personal journey, along with examples from her vast clinical experience, with compassionate insight and immediately actionable advice. This book is a must-read for anyone seeking to navigate the overlooked and misunderstood world of postpartum anxiety with resilience and hope."

> —**Layne Kumetz, MD**, obstetrician/gynecologist in Beverly Hills, CA;
> and attending physician at Cedars Sinai Medical Center

"*Hello Baby, Goodbye Intrusive Thoughts* is a must-read for new mothers silently battling anxiety, worries, or OCD. Jenny Yip compassionately explores the intersection of motherhood and intrusive thoughts, providing invaluable insights and evidence-based strategies to navigate this often-isolating experience. From tackling the unique challenges of the postpartum period to dissecting societal pressures fostering perfectionism and guilt, this is an essential companion for anyone on the profound journey of motherhood."

> —**Sabine Wilhelm, PhD**, professor at Harvard Medical School, and director
> of the Center for OCD and Related Disorders (CORD) at Massachusetts
> General Hospital

"Jenny Yip's book would have saved me so much strife over a decade ago as a new parent with OCD. I'm thrilled that people who give birth and their families can now turn to *Hello Baby, Goodbye Intrusive Thoughts*. From guiding readers through embracing uncertainty to coaching them on how to let go of socially constructed pressure put on new moms, this book is a game changer for parents with anxiety."

> —**Kavin Senapathy**, science and health journalist, and author of
> *The Progressive Parent*

"Jenny Yip has opened up about her own struggles with OCD in a way that will resonate with many. For years, people have turned to her for guidance as a specialist on OCD. This book will continue to solidify her as a go-to person in this field, and will also serve as a road map to help many other mothers with their own struggles."

> —**Stephanie Siegel**, founder of S Media-Consulting, and former supervising
> producer for NBC News

"Jenny Yip's book on OCD is a beacon of hope for families navigating this complex journey. Her insightful, compassionate approach has transformed the way my family understands, navigates, and dare I say, 'cured' OCD. Yip's expertise shines through every page, offering practical tools and empowering insights. This book is a must for anyone touched by OCD. Yip has profoundly impacted our healing journey and deep understanding about OCD. She's true magic."

—**Jennifer Meyer,** CEO and founder of Jennifer Meyer Jewelry

"In *Hello Baby, Goodbye Intrusive Thoughts*, Jenny Yip brings to light an often-overlooked aspect of motherhood. This book is a vital resource for expecting parents, unraveling the complexities of intrusive thoughts and the guilt they bring. Its honest and insightful approach makes it a must-read for navigating the emotional landscape of motherhood. I wholeheartedly recommend it as a guide to reclaiming wellness and joy in the journey of parenting."

—**Jonathan S. Abramowitz, PhD,** professor, and director of clinical training at the University of North Carolina at Chapel Hill

"Jenny Yip explores the perinatal territory of women's experiences with negative intrusive thoughts by sharing her personal experience and through the stories of other women. This is a very emotionally powerful, engaging book that will reach women who silently suffer, wondering if they are alone in struggling with the challenges and shame that OCD, postpartum depression, and/or anxiety brings. Yip provides wise guidance and practical strategies."

—**Barbara Van Noppen, PhD, LCSW,** clinical professor of psychiatry and the behavioral sciences, and vice chair for faculty development at the Keck School of Medicine at the University of Southern California

"Practical and compelling answers for new moms on how to navigate through the often-overwhelming anxiety, OCD, and depression that can strike after childbirth. Jenny Yip's honest stories of her struggles with OCD, along with her experience as a clinician, bring the book alive and provide hope for these common mental health challenges—so that everyone in the family can shed debilitating worry and get back to bonding with baby!"

—**Susan Boaz,** board president of the International OCD Foundation, and passionate advocate for everyone with OCD

HELLO BABY, GOODBYE INTRUSIVE THOUGHTS

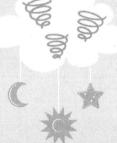

**Stop the Spiral of Anxiety & OCD to Reclaim
Wellness on Your Motherhood Journey**

Jenny Yip, PsyD

New Harbinger Publications, Inc.

NEW HARBINGER PUBLICATIONS is a registered trademark of New Harbinger Publications, Inc.

New Harbinger Publications is an employee-owned company.

Copyright © 2024 by Jenny Yip
New Harbinger Publications, Inc.
5720 Shattuck Avenue
Oakland, CA 94609
www.newharbinger.com

Cover design by Sara Christian

Acquired by Ryan Buresh

Edited by Diedre Hammons

Library of Congress Cataloging-in-Publication Data on file

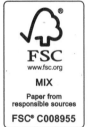

Printed in the United States of America

26   25   24

10   9   8   7   6   5   4   3   2   1   First Printing

For all mothers.

Contents

Part I

WHY DO WE GET ANXIOUS AND FRIGHTENING THOUGHTS?

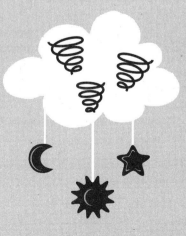

Introduction

Having Intrusive Thoughts Doesn't Mean You're a Bad Mom

My Experience

I went into labor with twin boys at thirty-eight weeks already knowing that Baby A was breached. Tristan was in the exact same position since the second trimester and hadn't bothered turning around. I was ready for a cesarean delivery, and didn't actually mind it. Trying to push two six-pound babies out of my vagina seemed a whole lot worse. My husband put on my yoga meditative music in the labor room where my phenomenal OB greeted me with a reassuring smile. Soon after receiving the epidural, a blue drape slid across me, hanging over my chest as the nurses helped me lie back down. Then I just waited patiently while the skilled medical team worked their magic to bring me my babies. The miracle of finally meeting my precious boys after dreaming of them for nine whole months was a feeling no words could describe.

My husband stayed by my side, holding my anxiously awaiting hands as he watched each baby over the drape be pulled out of my ginormous belly. I heard my boys' first cries while the medical team assessed each baby's post-delivery condition before they were ready to be in my eager arms. Baby B was cleared first even though he was delivered a few minutes after. I was over the moon, welling up with joyful tears to finally meet Dash. I held him dearly against my skin, unaware of the commotion happening on the other side. My husband left our side to check on the situation, running interference between the needs of his newborn sons on either side of that drape. Then the pediatric team announced they were rushing Tristan to the NICU for respiratory support.

I was dumbfounded. What's wrong with Tristan? Where were they taking my baby? I hadn't even had a glance at him. What I wasn't ready for that day was not having both of my sweet loves in my arms after delivery. All of a sudden, a dark cloud of dread swirled over me. Still paralyzed from anesthesia, I felt helpless and powerless. I couldn't just get up and run after them wheeling my baby away. Everyone who remained in the labor room kept reassuring me that everything would be fine. I tried to believe them. I tried to focus my attention and adoration on the baby in my arms. "At least I have Dash here with me," I kept telling myself, tricking my brain to look at the positives. However, the floodgate of tragic images was already unlocked and raided my mind with unimaginable catastrophic fears.

"What if Tristan isn't able to breathe on his own and the medical team can't help him? What if something worse is happening and he's now suffering terribly? What if he dies before I even get to see him and I never get to hold or experience his little body in my arms? What if Dash feels his missing twin and has to live a life always feeling this emptiness?"

These images and thoughts swept my imagination into a tornado of fears. Anguish at myself soon followed for even having such terrible, pessimistic thoughts. "What kind of mother would have such tragic thoughts of her newborn?" My mind quickly sank deeper and deeper into panic mode and I was no longer present with Dash. Yet, somewhere along the spiral of anxiety, I was taken aback by the familiarity of the frightening intrusive thoughts that reminded me of the constant dread I had felt the first half of my life. The content was now different, though that peculiar feeling of terror was undeniably familiar.

Having battled obsessive-compulsive disorder (OCD) since the age of four, finally triumphing over it in my twenties and later becoming a specialist in treating the most severe cases of OCD, I was shocked at the devastating effect OCD had on me once again. Not only was I overly arrogant that I had defeated OCD for good, the thought of experiencing OCD postpartum never even crossed my mind. Surely, I had treated many women suffering from perinatal OCD and anxiety. And like most people having overcome OCD, I had minor intrusive thoughts here and there that were now easily ignored. However, being deeply trapped in relentless images of potential harm to my loved ones along with silly magical compulsions to ensure their safety were things of the past—so I thought. I was wrong. OCD tackles whatever it is that you care about, especially when you least expect it. In that moment, what I cared deeply about was the health and safety of my twin babies.

Still, I didn't realize OCD had taken over again. It wasn't until I confided in a mentor about my struggles being a new mom that she suggested the possibility of OCD. There it was—my OCD was clever as ever, disguising itself in nebulous form. Even I, the OCD specialist, could not see it. It had become even trickier than I ever remembered with dreadful intrusive thoughts and magical safety rituals that were more creative and obscure. That was how my OCD monster tugged at my heartstrings and kept me hostage to its senseless rules during my initial postpartum days. All in the guise of keeping my babies safe, paradoxically so. In reality, my baby-mother bond was far from safe with OCD hanging around.

Having intrusive, frightening thoughts doesn't mean you're a bad mother. Trust me. I've been there. It's actually quite the opposite. This is because intrusive thoughts are unwelcomed, involuntary ideas or images that intrude into your mind without your conscious intent, permission, or control. These thoughts tend to consist of disturbing, socially inappropriate, or worrisome content against your personal values and beliefs, paving the way for your anxiety to spiral. Consequently, our anxiety monster will tackle whatever we intensely care about. If you're concerned about being a morally righteous person—BOOM, you'll question your every action and worry that you're not meeting the ethical standards of motherhood. If you care about how others perceive your character as a mom, then your antennae will constantly be alert to others' reactions as you worry about what people say, do, or how they look at you.

Whether you're a new or veteran mom, contemplating pregnancy, or in your postpartum period, intrusive frightening thoughts and worries can impact your choices and motherhood journey if you let them. You might consider becoming a mother for the first time and be influenced by endless worries about the risks and stresses of pregnancy. When you are pregnant, your mind might be bombarded by intrusive fears of all of the potential health threats to you and baby. If you're a new mom finally meeting your little one whom you've protected in your belly for nine whole months, you just might have frighteningly shattering thoughts of all the possible harm that can come to your helpless newborn. You have these terrifyingly disturbing thoughts not because you're a terrible person or a bad mother. You have such frightening intrusive thoughts because you care profoundly about your loving baby.

The stressors of motherhood are challenging enough without the intrusive thoughts and worries that often raise doubt about our mothering capabilities. Truth is, when we enter our motherhood journey, we tend to devote our entire beings to our children and family while automatically sacrificing our individual identity and needs for wellness. Out of our natural instincts to care and protect our baby, we give and give and give. Yet, at the drop of a pin, when we believe we've failed to meet the expectations of motherhood, we're quick to perceive ourselves as a bad mom while we strive even harder to live up to society's supermom ideals. Hence, whatever we do never seems enough, and eventually, however much we do, we might still believe that we aren't enough. And so, in this unjustified perspective lies the source for our alarming intrusive thoughts and worries.

To reclaim your wellness throughout your motherhood journey, you have to stop the spiral of anxiety by making room for the uncertainties of real life. My job is to provide you with the awareness and strategies to be empowered to do this hard work while honoring your maternal wellness. In these chapters, you'll learn how the burdens of our mothering roles without adequate wellness contribute to intrusive, frightening thoughts and worries. You'll grasp how avoiding your fears actually reinforce their intensity and acquire valuable tools to reduce their consequential effects. You'll cultivate a flexible mindset focused on resiliency for both you and baby, enabling you to let go of unnecessary worries and anxiety. You'll rediscover the value of your new mom identity and recognize the significance of emplacing healthy boundaries to protect your authentic bond with your baby and family. Most importantly, you'll realize that striving for perfection in your motherhood journey is the culprit for stress and unwellness.

The strategies within these chapters will be highlighted by various stories. Remi will underscore the stressful questions and concerns that she struggled with in the preconception stage. You'll hear how Kendall prevailed over her intrusive thoughts and fears of inadequacy during her prenatal period after two previous miscarriages. Madelyn will highlight the paradoxical consequences of avoidance that contributed to feelings of failure and self-doubt as she confronted postpartum anxiety and depression. You'll get insight into how Wilmina, with a young toddler at hand and a baby on the way, shifted her mindset from anxious thoughts of perfectionism, worries, and guilt to enforce long-term wellness. In addition, I'll also continue to share my battles with intrusive thoughts from my OCD monster during the postpartum period. The intricate nature of each of these stories may or may not relate to your particular intrusive thoughts or worries. Nevertheless, my hope is to provide context to how you can utilize each strategy in your own journey to defeat your anxious monster.

By flexing your mental muscles and practicing the tools within these pages, you'll begin to create new habits that will honor your boundaries and well-being as a new mama. Rather than constantly feeling intensely anxious from intrusive thoughts of harm to your little love or being paralyzed by irrational doubts of your capability, imagine your motherhood journey free from such nonsense mind traps. It's possible.

I reclaimed my mind from the spiral of anxiety, motivated by love for my babies. Using the strategies provided in this book, you too can stop the spiral of anxiety as you reclaim wellness on your motherhood journey.

Chapter 1

The Truth About "Maternal Wellness"

Maternal wellness—what does it mean to you? In the healthcare community, it refers to the physical, emotional, and mental well-being of mothers, especially during the perinatal period. It focuses on the necessary aspects to a mother's health, such as having essential healthcare services, stress management, adequate rest and nutrition, and proper resources to support a mother's role and responsibilities to her children and family. However, throughout a woman's motherhood journey, the actual reality is far from that ideal, and this is especially evidenced in the early days. Even with the advances in today's world, many mothers still face challenges accessing maternal healthcare. From preconception onward, the truth is that maternal wellness is overlooked and disregarded, leading many women to feel neglected.

Aside from the basic needs and support systems that are lacking to maintain a mother's wellness, there are also unrealistic societal expectations imposed on mothers for them to prioritize their family's needs above their own well-being. Even in a two-parent home, the disparity in childcare and household demands between mothers and fathers is discouraging. On top of it all, the invisible responsibilities placed on mothers, such as having to coordinate all things related to running a household, become so time-consuming and emotionally exhausting that they often lead to anxiety, depression, burnout, and poor overall health. Yet, because of the double standards, gender stereotypes, and societal pressures for mothers to do it all, we consequently feel inadequate, guilty, and shameful when we fail to meet these unsustainable expectations.

In this discrepancy between what we're expected to achieve and what we're realistically able to sustain lies the playground for intrusive, frightening thoughts. Negative feelings of guilt, shame, and fear of all the ways that we could be inadequate mothers and all the things that could harm our loved ones provide the natural fuel for our anxiety monster to taunt us with disturbing worries. Additionally, when such intrusive dreaded thoughts take over our minds, we believe that we must be at fault and further blame our imperfect selves for allowing this to happen. No wonder many mothers, especially new moms, are constantly spiraling in anxiety, daunting worries, and self-doubt.

To break this vicious, lopsided cycle, we have to make space for our mothering flaws and build compassion for the imperfect realities of motherhood. We have to acknowledge not just the inequities that exist in societal expectations; we have to also address expectations for ourselves and each other if we want to kick our anxious monster to the curb. To truly promote maternal wellness, we cannot persist in neglecting our individual needs only to be of service to our families and communities. We must begin to emphasize and value ourselves by asserting healthy boundaries and advocating for our own personal wellness.

At any point in our maternal role, intrusive frightening thoughts can attack our well-being if we let them, especially when unrealistic expectations pile on. Or we can acknowledge the untenable societal pressures and learn to change our own irrational narratives that keep us stuck. To ascertain how our senseless expectations can make way for anxiety and upsetting intrusive thoughts, let's meet Remi, Kendall, Madelyn, and Wilmina—each woman at various stages of motherhood, from preconception to postpartum and beyond.

Preconception: Remi

> Remi left her OB appointment for her annual check feeling more confused
> than before arriving. At the tender age of thirty, she grappled with the
> difficult decision of whether to start a family or continue to pursue her
> passions in journalism. Like so many women in her cohort, the double
> standards and societal pressures to be both professionally driven and
> remain family-oriented seemed doable yet somehow untenable. Her
> husband of two years had been very supportive of her career and her
> timeline despite desperately wanting to start their own family. However,
> Remi didn't think her biological timeline was as compassionate. Several of
> her single colleagues had frozen their eggs for later use when a mate
> became available. Remi, on the other hand, wasn't waiting for a mate.
> She simply wasn't sure when would be the right time to have a baby and
> start their family. Inspired by the superwoman powers depicted in her
> social media feeds, Remi had high expectations of herself to take on both
> motherhood and careerhood equally. Yet, since nothing in her earlier years
> really prepared her for these preconception questions, she felt anxiously
> vulnerable and unprepared to make such permanent life decisions.

Like Remi, many women wish they'd had a conversation about maternal
wellness before even attempting pregnancy. That's because pregnancy is
only possible during a small window of time in a woman's life, and depending on various circumstances, your decision will have a direct impact on
the how, when, where, and what's of your motherhood journey if you
choose that path. For example, the timing of your decision to start a family
will often determine whether you'll be able to conceive naturally or require
fertility treatments. If you tend to be a worrier and ruminate over every
catastrophic consequence whenever faced with big life decisions, then
having little knowledge of family planning or fertility options available to
you will likely fuel your anxiety monster.

As it turns out, many young women are uninformed about the available
choices and resources related to pregnancy and feel ill-equipped to handle
the stresses of motherhood, causing fear and anxiety (Declercq et al. 2002).
In fact, an estimated 50 percent of pregnancies in the United States are
still unplanned (Aztlan-James, McLemore, and Taylor 2017). Without the

necessary support, awareness, and open conversations regardless of age or life circumstances, you may feel apprehensive and uncomfortable making decisions related to your reproductive health and family planning goals. Moreover, depending on your cultural upbringing, which comes with various expectations, the decision to prioritize or delay pregnancy can be an additional source of anxiety and unrest in your personal fertility journey.

For instance, you may have been encouraged to pursue higher education or a professional career in your twenties and thirties instead of starting your own family. On the other hand, you may have also been expected to prioritize the care of your family or others over a career. Regardless of these conflicting expectations, the demands on a woman to balance the various gender-biased roles and responsibilities can result in significant pressure to be a professional, caregiver, and partner all at the same time. In fact, women have been shaped by societal expectations to be able to do it all, even though *doing it all* comes with a price tag.

The numerous roles we try to uphold with various undefined duties have led many women to exhaustion and burnout (Dunatchik and Speight 2020). Plus, when we fail to do it all or do it flawlessly, we tend to criticize and judge ourselves for not doing and being enough. Like Remi, you might've questioned your ability to handle motherhood. You might've even experienced imposter syndrome and concluded with such self-defeating narratives as *"If I can't do it perfectly, people will think I'm a fraud"* or *"I can't even keep up now. I'll never be able to juggle work and family as I'm expected to."*

Remember Rosie the Riveter, the iconic image of a strong woman flexing her biceps? Although Rosie was originally a symbol of women's empowerment in the workforce during World War II with her iconic "We Can Do It!" slogan, Rosie has since evolved and been adopted to represent the ability of women to excel in multiple roles with determination and strength that has become modern motherhood. This superwoman myth displayed in media has depicted highly successful women with impeccable appearances, perfect families, and spotless homes. These are all implicit messages that to be successful, a woman must effortlessly balance multiple demands, which sets an untenable standard for you to live by. If you, like Remi and most women, care to uphold these societal expectations yet struggle to do it effortlessly, then your mind will likely spiral with self-doubt and intrusive worries as you anxiously contemplate over such big life decisions as pregnancy.

On the other hand, if you choose to start your family later in life, infertility and other reproductive health issues can also make the preconception journey emotionally and physically difficult. Having one or more miscarriages often comes with feelings of guilt and an overwhelming sense of responsibility for the loss of pregnancy. Again, because of societal standards for us to be able to do it all, a woman may judge herself for struggling through this process, even if nothing could've prevented the loss. Your mind may be filled with intrusive thoughts of harm and inadequacies, creating further anxiety about future pregnancies and the possibility of another loss. Unfortunately, when we need our social support the most to remain well, societal shame and stigma often deter us from discussing the grief and pain we feel, steering many women to isolation and emotional disconnection during the preconception period.

The truth is that we live in a culture that places unrealistic expectations on women to do it all without adequate support or resources. The implicit messages that have shaped our beliefs of womanhood set us up for the spiral of anxious thoughts when we're unable to meet these exorbitant societal demands. To truly enhance a woman's physical, emotional, and mental wellness, changes have to start at the very beginning to provide the space for open, nonjudgmental dialogues about family planning, fertility options, and pregnancy struggles without senseless expectations from our minds.

Prenatal: Kendall

Kendall met each day with gratitude for having maintained her current pregnancy this far along. After two consecutive miscarriages and many emotional conflicts with her husband in the last few years, she had almost given up. Now in her second trimester, she was cautiously hopeful to finally have the family life she had dreamed of. Except, given her fertility history, she also felt constant apprehension about the possibility of another loss. Knowing her OB tended to give blunt feedback, Kendall anticipated every prenatal care appointment with spiraling anxiety about what her OB might say. After each visit, she worried for days about all the dos, don'ts, and what-to-watch-out-fors forewarned by her OB. Being well aware of Kendall's history with anxiety, her husband had urged her to take up meditation, breath work, and yoga to safeguard their pregnancy and mitigate stressors. However, Kendall still felt uneasy whenever she wasn't engaged in one of these calming exercises. She wanted to keep her focus on the positives instead of dwelling on the potential negatives, though didn't know what else to do to escape the uncomfortable thoughts that seemed to consume her entire being daily.

Kendall's experience of the mixed emotions that naturally come with pregnancy is not uncommon. Many parents envision the time from pregnancy to birth as an occasion for celebratory joy. Although this journey has its beautiful moments, it also takes a toll on a mother's well-being that can leave her with many foreign emotions and experiences. As you might imagine, pregnancy impacts your entire being—physically, emotionally, and mentally. However, aside from the regular prenatal appointments where attention toward the fetus is the main focus, little, if any, emphasis is placed on a mother's emotional or mental wellness (Firoz et al. 2018). Research has illustrated time and again that a woman's mental health during pregnancy has a direct impact on her baby's neurological development, fetal heart rate, and overall health (Scheinost et al. 2017). Yet, despite this knowledge, the true wellness of a mother as a whole person, independent from pregnancy, is still often neglected and unacknowledged.

Just as Kendall experienced, this period is naturally met with fear and anxiety for many new moms. Your concerns about the health of baby, discomforts brought on by drastic hormonal fluctuations, fears of miscarriage, and apprehension about the pains from delivery are just a few of numerous sources for worries and anxiety. However, few obstetricians provide unrushed opportunities during prenatal *wellness* visits to address such concerns so you feel heard, regarded, and understood. In fact, if you've felt unreasonably judged, pressured, or scared while being prodded and examined by a disapproving doctor who was more concerned about what you were doing right or wrong for baby's physical health than your own wellness, you are not alone. Many of my patients have expressed discouragement after leaving prenatal care appointments, feeling like a medical subject containing a highly valued scientific specimen.

Another common frustration voiced by numerous new mothers whom I've guided through the prenatal period is the societal gender bias that places the inconvenience of prenatal changes as solely the woman's responsibility. For instance, even though Kendall's husband was helpful to suggest resources, few expectant fathers adjust their lifestyle during the prenatal period or have the empathic understanding of the demands of pregnancy to truly be a compassionate support system for their partners. Mothers often feel misunderstood and alone as they're expected to continue their regular daily responsibilities atop of all the physical, emotional, and mental fluctuations from pregnancy. If your partner demonstrates a lack of participation, attention, or affection, or becomes dismissive, unresponsive, or insensitive during this vulnerable period, the emotional disconnect will surely add further stress on your motherhood journey. Without the proper education and resources for both mothers and partners, many couples often find themselves in conflict with one another before baby is even born.

If you tend to be a worrier like Kendall, pregnancy serves as the optimal time for your anxiety monster to fill your mind with intrusive, catastrophic thoughts. You might ruminate about harm to baby or yourself during your pregnancy and delivery. You might worry incessantly about getting adequate nutrition, avoiding toxic environments, potential birth defects, or congenital health conditions. You might fear miscarrying or even maternal illness and death. While a mild level of these concerns is to be expected, excessive doubt about your ability to handle the physical, emotional, and mental demands of motherhood can be debilitating without a comprehensive supportive system in place to ensure true maternal wellness.

Given the importance of your mental, emotional, and physical health, it's imperative to empower yourself with available education and resources, while eliminating unnecessary expectations and judgments of yourself during your prenatal experience. Engage your partner and close family or friends in open communications to feel heard, understood, and validated. Ask your healthcare provider for additional support if needed. Believe it or not, you can take charge of your overall well-being before, during, or after pregnancy. Putting irrational expectations and criticizing self-narratives aside will give you a chance to dive deeper into your own wellness as a whole.

Postpartum: Madelyn

Madelyn held her newborn to her left breast and gently caressed her baby's cheek to get him to latch. It was just about midnight, and she was giving a final feeding before handing her baby over to her night doula for the next five hours. She knew being a single mother would have its challenges, especially being a new mom. Regardless, the exhaustion and brain fog she felt from having to keep up a two-to-three-hour feeding schedule for the past two weeks was incomparable to anything she had ever experienced. Despite her due diligence in carefully planning for the baby's arrival and her recovery, she didn't feel as prepared as she expected to be. In fact, Madelyn found herself in a constant state of restlessness, questioning every decision she had made. When her pediatrician inquired about her adjustment to new motherhood at a baby wellness visit, Madelyn confided that she no longer felt like herself. She was doubtful of her mothering capability and frequently irritable given her seeming inability to bond with her baby. Her pediatrician acknowledged that her experiences were a normal part of the baby blues and that things would improve in the weeks ahead. Despite this reassurance, Madelyn was skeptical and couldn't recall any positive feelings since giving birth. She didn't know what happened to that initial excitement when she held her baby for the very first time. However, she definitely didn't want to feel the dread that had hung over her since bringing baby home.

The birth of a baby is indeed a celebratory occasion for many new parents, extended family, and friends. The joy of seeing and holding your newborn is an ecstatic feeling incomparable to any others. Though, following the initial bliss comes the recovery and adjustment of caring for a new, defenseless human that can at times lead to anxiety and depression for some new moms, as in Madelyn's case. Medically, pregnancy consists of three trimesters; however, some have identified the postpartum period as a "fourth trimester," recognized for its "critical transition period with unmet maternal health needs" (Firoz et al. 2018). The postpartum journey is not only a process of physical healing for a mother, it is also a period for learning to adapt to a new life with a newborn. During this period of adjustment, you might experience many high highs along with many low lows that can leave you with unfamiliar and overwhelming emotions.

In fact, whether you deliver vaginally, by cesarean, in a hospital maternity ward, or by a doula in a more comfortable environment, care and attention provided to a new mother after the birthing process is very short-lived. As a new mom, you're expected to quickly bring your newborn home and be responsible for another life without having any skills or previous experience. You're expected to rapidly adjust to caring for a baby and all their needs while being stuck with limited mobility and physical injury from deep labor incisions. You're expected to immediately breastfeed, be a pro at doing so, and keep up a feeding schedule of every two to three hours for the initial weeks, regardless of your body's exhaustion and needs for recovery. On top of it all, you're expected to be overjoyed despite your mental fog, physical fatigue, or the swift hormonal changes that can cause contradictory feelings of anxiety and depression. Like Madelyn, these expectations have left many new mothers feeling uneasy, lost, and even less supported, paving the way for unhealthy intrusive thoughts. In reality, none of this reflects maternal wellness, and instead, creates the perfect storm for postpartum *unwellness*.

Madelyn, for instance, was experiencing postpartum anxiety and depression. Although, like many new moms, she didn't know how to get appropriate help. In fact, a significant proportion of mothers who experience perinatal mental illness often go undiagnosed, leaving many to suffer from anxiety, depression, obsessive-compulsive disorder (OCD), or even psychosis during this vulnerable time. Effective maternal mental health treatments are indeed available and can literally be lifesaving to protect the well-being of both mother and baby. However, stigma, lack of awareness, misdiagnosis, and limited routine screenings all continue to be barriers to accessing proper care. While early identification and treatment can prevent more severe symptoms, the truth is few new mothers are given adequate attention and care, and even fewer are assessed for postpartum symptoms (Firoz et al. 2018).

All things considered, encouraging compassionate dialogues about maternal mental health can greatly improve early detection and provide the emotional support needed by so many mothers. Although research related to perinatal mental illness remains limited, it's worthwhile to take a closer look at the ones most talked about today. If you recognize these symptoms in your own motherhood journey, it's crucial for you to seek professional guidance from a mental healthcare provider experienced in treating perinatal conditions.

Perinatal Depression

Even with a support system and resources, many new mothers often feel overwhelmed and left behind, which can lead to emotional isolation and a heightened risk for postpartum mental illness. In fact, although some women are regularly screened for and educated about postpartum depression at prenatal and postnatal care visits, many are not. Postpartum depression isn't just the blues after giving birth. It's a common mood disorder that affects around 10 to 15 percent of new mothers worldwide, especially in the absence of resources and a strong supportive network (Anokye et al. 2018). Sadly, the proportion of mothers impacted is likely much higher given the number of women who are un- or misdiagnosed. Symptoms include a wide range of emotions like sadness, irritability, anxiety, and feelings of guilt or worthlessness. Common thoughts you might have if you're suffering from postpartum depression sound like, "I feel overwhelmed and hopeless." "I'm not enjoying motherhood and don't feel connected with my baby." Or "I'm a burden on my family and don't feel like myself anymore." Regardless of your income, race, or social status, know that you are not alone in this experience—perinatal depression impacts many mothers, new and veteran.

Perinatal Anxiety

While stress and anxiety are common experiences for many new parents, debilitating anxiety can persist for as many as 11 to 21 percent of mothers (Dubber et al. 2015). Again, since this estimate comes only from diagnosed cases, postpartum anxiety is another common condition that likely affects many more mothers. Symptoms can include excessive worries and racing thoughts about the health and safety of baby and self, as well as uneasy physical bodily symptoms like heart palpitations or shortness of breath. A new mom experiencing postpartum anxiety may constantly question her own abilities to care for her baby such as, "What if something bad happens to my baby?" "I'm not doing a good enough job as a mother" or "I can't handle this." You might question whether you're meeting expectations— your own and that of others. You might also seek reassurances from others like a performance review to ensure everything is perfect. Perinatal anxiety also doesn't discriminate and can negatively impact your motherhood journey regardless of your race or socioeconomic status. Unfortunately, since much more attention has been placed on perinatal depression, those mothers who experience perinatal anxiety and seek help are often misdiagnosed and only treated for depression.

Perinatal Obsessive-Compulsive Disorder

At a more intense level, when intrusive ruminations involve unwanted and often frightening thoughts or images of harm or catastrophic consequences to baby accompanied by compulsive and sometimes magical safety behaviors, these symptoms warrant a diagnosis of postpartum obsessive-compulsive disorder (OCD). Common intrusive OCD thoughts you might have during this period include, "What if I accidentally harm or even drown my baby?" "The milk bottle could be poisoned with chemicals unless I follow a strict sanitizing routine." "I must stay and watch my infant while she sleeps to prevent SIDS." Intrusive OCD thoughts elicit an urgency to do something to circumvent the feared disastrous outcome in order to gain temporary relief. Hence, you feel the need to repeat the compulsions whenever the thoughts arise despite feeling the absurdity of the behaviors. Again, postpartum OCD doesn't discriminate, and it's unclear how common it is due to the lack of awareness and research. However, some estimates claim as many as 10 to 50 percent of new mothers actually suffer from postpartum OCD, which is often misdiagnosed as depression (Ali 2018).

Although less common compared to mothers, postpartum OCD can also affect new fathers. This new area of research has found approximately 1 to 2.3 percent of fathers develop symptoms, which are similar to those experienced by mothers (Walker et al. 2021). Fathers who feel isolated or lack a strong social and emotional support system are at higher risk for intrusive thoughts related to harm, safety, and health to baby along with compulsive checking, cleaning, or handwashing. Previous experience of OCD, anxiety, or perfectionistic tendencies are also risk factors as well as difficulty adjusting to the responsibility and stress of becoming a new parent. Regardless, whether symptoms develop in mothers or fathers, onset tends to be intense and appear out of the blue. Additionally, many new parents fear disclosing their symptoms due to their offensive nature, social stigma, and the possible negative consequence of having their baby removed. In fact, postpartum OCD is often confused with postpartum psychosis even by medical and mental health professionals. Nevertheless, finding a mental healthcare professional experienced in treating OCD is imperative to alleviating symptoms during this critical bonding period.

Perinatal Psychosis

While postpartum OCD involves unwanted, intrusive thoughts of potential harm to baby accompanied by irrational, magical reactions to prevent the feared outcome, the thoughts and images are unwanted and don't fit with your belief system. On the other hand, a new mom suffering from postpartum psychosis cannot differentiate her delusional thoughts from reality. You may have thoughts such as, "I hear voices that I'm not in control of and am unsure what's real or not" "My baby is in danger unless I harm myself to protect him." Or "I must remove my child from the threats of this world to save her soul." Postpartum psychosis is a rare yet serious mental health illness affecting about 0.1 to 0.2 percent of women and involves hallucinations, disordered thinking, mania, confusion, and paranoia (Işık 2018). Women with a history of bipolar disorder, schizophrenia, or other psychotic disorders are at higher risk. Since a mother suffering from postpartum psychosis cannot tell whether her thoughts are truly her own, it's a medical emergency presenting potentially grave risk to both mother and baby. Hence, seeking immediate support from a healthcare professional is vital and can be lifesaving.

Clearly, women with a lack of resources or social support are at an increased risk for suffering from postpartum illness overall. Whether a new mom experiences postpartum depression, anxiety, OCD, or psychosis, one common denominator remains constant across all postpartum mental illness—it interferes with a mother's ability to care for herself, her baby, or bond with her newborn. In fact, if you feel a reluctance to disclose your symptoms or ask for help out of fear of societal stigma, being viewed as a bad mother, or being separated from baby, you are not alone. Nevertheless, neglecting these symptoms and your wellness will ultimately give your anxiety monster permission to terrorize you with disturbing intrusive thoughts.

Aside from mental health concerns during the postpartum period, few mothers, including Madelyn, have felt supported to handle the multitude of baby care and daily household responsibilities. Without sufficient time to care for yourself, it is easy to lose your identity during the initial postpartum days and weeks. Add the mental and physical fatigue to the mix for having to care for a newborn 24/7 can quickly lead you to feelings of failure, inadequacy, worthlessness, guilt, disconnection, isolation, and suffocation. All of which fuel daunting intrusive thoughts instead of honoring your maternal wellness.

Toddlerhood & Beyond: Wilmina

When Wilmina learned that she was pregnant with their second child, her initial reaction was mixed. Being overextended with their first child who had just turned a year old and already exhibiting full-blown tantrums, she wrestled with the reality of having another child so soon. Even though her husband was very involved in childcare and prioritized their family over his work or social commitments, Wilmina aspired to be THE supermom yet still grappled to perfectly balance motherhood and her career.

Now pregnant again, her mind constantly spiraled to anxiety about her struggles as a new mom with their first pregnancy. Not only was it a challenging time for her physically, she also battled relentless intrusive thoughts and worries, and now feared their return. Believing she had already lost her mind with one child, she had a hard time fathoming having two. She wished her firstborn was already walking and talking efficiently to give her a bit more flexibility and confidence to handle the responsibilities of another child. Rather, she imagined a bazillion "what if" scenarios, and each was followed by more worries. Instead of feeling the excitement that her husband displayed, Wilmina felt guilt and shame for having such dreaded thoughts and wondered when these alarming worries would finally ease up. Alas, being unable to contain these uncomfortable feelings or pinpoint why she felt this way left her feeling even more perplexed and anxious.

Many mothers I've helped have wondered whether it'll get better—whether their intrusive distressing thoughts and worries will ever go away. I won't lie. Without adequate support and resources, ongoing mothering obligations will continue to compromise the idea of maternal wellness as your children age. You'll still get worrisome thoughts simply because you care deeply about your little one. The thoughts will just shift with your motherhood journey as you adapt to different challenges according to your child's development. Like Wilmina, you might be anxiously anticipating baby to walk and talk. Yet, when they finally start walking, your mind might be filled with a new set of catastrophic fears of all the dangers they could get into. Similarly, when they start talking and begin screaming bloody murder at you one day, you might be stunned with self-doubt while ruminating over all the ways you've failed as a parent. Someone once said, you'll spend the first two years of your child's life teaching them to walk and talk, and the next sixteen telling them to sit down and be quiet.

Without missing a beat, I've been my twin boys' most beloved mama *and* hated villain all at the same time. They don't call it the terrible twos, thunderous threes, and effing fours for no reason. During the toddler years, you might worry and wonder what happened to your angelic baby who's suddenly become a dramatic tyrant. You might feel like you've lost your mind as you anxiously attempt to circumvent every emotional meltdown. Your mind might spiral with upsetting intrusive thoughts of what you're doing wrong during these overwhelming moments. Then, when you add another child to the picture, as in Wilmina's case, you might ruminate over all of the dreaded possibilities from having to balance it all.

Yes, you will continue to have intrusive, worrisome thoughts—because we all do. Yet, just because you have such thoughts and worries doesn't mean you have to be held hostage by them, and your wellness doesn't have to remain an illusory concept. Whenever your core becomes filled with guilt, shame, or inadequacy as you ruminate about a brainless mistake, possible harm to baby, or the things you could've done differently, just know it's your anxious monster at play.

To genuinely ensure maternal wellness, you have to prioritize your own physical, emotional, and mental health. Even though society expects mothers to be everything and everywhere at the drop of a hat, it doesn't mean you have to maintain that perfect facade and live up to the supermom pressures that Wilmina and many mothers aspire to. Instead, value your own needs and individual identities separate from just a selfless caretaker. Assert healthy boundaries and instill values free from societal gender stereotypes. Drop the superwoman image that the world expects mothers to live up to. Not that you're not strong—you most definitely are as exemplified in all that you already do and carry. It's just unrealistic and unhealthy to expect yourself to be strong 100 percent of the time. At the end of the day, your value is much more significant than the superficial impression of supermom.

Having this awareness of the various circumstances that can compromise maternal wellness gives you a starting framework for how dreaded intrusive thoughts and worries often arise. As you read the following chapters, you'll begin to move toward maternal wellness by practicing the skills offered. Rather than hopelessly resisting or futilely reacting to your persistent anxiety monster, you'll learn what you can do instead. Along your motherhood journey, consider each anxious moment as a direct opportunity to learn from and to transform your experience using the tools you'll acquire within these pages.

With more compassion and less self-judgment, there will also be fewer opportunities for intrusive alarming thoughts to rob you and baby of wellness. As it turns out, maternal wellness doesn't just impact mothers individually; our well-being or lack of also directly affects our families and communities. Together, we can reclaim wellness by learning to navigate the rollercoaster of motherhood from preconception onwards.

Chapter 2

Don't Think of the Yellow Duck—Whatever You Resist Persists

Have you ever wondered why diets often fail? No matter what diet you've tried, you probably had a list of foods to stay away from. To be aware of the foods that you're *not* supposed to consume will require you to pay special attention to each sinful item. In turn, increasing your attention only heightens your thoughts around the foods that you're to avoid. Simply stated, it's a catch-22 that sabotages our efforts.

In truth, whatever you resist persists, whether it's foods or frightening intrusive thoughts. If avoiding a specific thought, your baby drowning, for example, only magnifies its content, would the opposite work to reduce its intensity? To grasp this concept and reclaim wellness from your anxious monster, you'll have to fully comprehend why resisting intrusive anxious thoughts is an unproductive strategy and what to do instead. First, let's understand how our thoughts, emotions, and behaviors are intertwined and affect one another.

Most Everything Is Out of Our Control

We have three very basic foundations to our functioning: our thoughts, emotions, and behaviors. Of the three, only one is within our direct control while we have zero direct control over the others. The three together influence what we think, how we feel, and what we do, and determine whether our intrusive worries and thoughts get louder or quieter. To start, we'll examine our thoughts and test whether you have direct control over them.

Thoughts

I want you to do a thinking experiment with me. Right now, close your eyes for a minute and don't think of the yellow duck. Really, don't think of the yellow duck. Now, don't think of the yellow duck in the blue pond. Next, don't think of the yellow duck in the blue pond next to the green tree. Try as you may, you likely still had a glimpse of the yellow duck, blue pond, and green tree even though the instructions were to not think about them. *Why does this occur?* you may wonder.

At any given second, we have billions of stimuli that enter and exit our awareness because of our five senses. Babies in the womb typically develop the senses of touch, taste, smell, hearing, and sight by the twenty-eighth week. From the moment these sensory inputs are established, they remain active twenty-four hours a day; absorbing information from the environment that forms thoughts to help us navigate and make sense of our world. We have no way of shutting off our five senses, not even in our sleep. We can plug our ears and still hear sounds. We can cover our eyes and still visualize images. These sensory inputs are constantly receiving billions of stimuli without a shut-off valve, many of which are out of our conscious awareness.

Close your eyes again and observe all of the different sounds, images, tactile sensations, even smells and tastes around you that you may not have previously noticed. This is called *selective attention*—your ability to choose the elements to focus on. Thus, even though you have no direct control over the type of thoughts you have because of your sensory inputs that operate without stop, what you do have control over is how you attend to the thoughts that you selectively dial in to. This is why attempting to *not* think of the yellow duck only encourages it. Any attempt to resist something is actually added energy and effort provided to the resistance.

On the other hand, what happens when you attempt to only think of the yellow duck and nothing else? Try it—*yellow duck, yellow duck, yellow duck, yellow duck, yellowduck, yellowduck, yellowduck, yellowduckyellowduck...* Eventually, that yellow duck starts to blur with other images simply because your mind gets bored over time when there are billions of other stimuli demanding your attention. This is the paradox of our thoughts, whether it's sinful chocolate-covered strawberries or alarming dreaded images of harm to our loved ones. Whatever we resist persists. Just the pure attempt to resist something adds volume to the thing itself to be resisted.

This paradox is also how intrusive, frightening thoughts can become so powerful. We have no direct control over the type of thoughts we have unless we purposefully conjure up specific thoughts that we selectively attend to. When thoughts arise seemingly out of the blue with content that we deem as forbidden or appalling, our initial reaction is often to push the thoughts out of our minds. However, this attempt only adds energy to the thought and magnifies its weight. Many moms have tried to escape unwanted thoughts of harm to baby, then blame themselves for the failed effort after trying the same unhelpful avoidance. In reality, each concerted effort to dismiss such dreaded thoughts only places more attention onto it, resulting in an unproductive cycle that actually paves the way for our anxiety monster to evolve and grow in strength.

Emotions

As it turns out, whatever we think, we feel. Just like thoughts, we also have no direct control over our emotions. We can attempt to suppress, deny, distract, or avoid our feelings; however, none of these methods directly control how and what we feel. This is because emotions are triggered from thoughts. Unless you possess some magical powers, simply snapping your fingers or waving a wand won't automatically change what you currently feel. To feel joy, you have to either be in an experience that conjures up joyous thoughts or reflect back on a past event that was interpreted as joyful. Similarly, to feel anger, you have to either be in a situation that evokes thoughts of injustice or be reminded of a past event where injustice was perceived. Emotional experiences are elicited from thoughts whether the thought occurs within your conscious awareness or not.

Being a new mom with unbalanced hormones rapidly rising and falling, your emotional state is a delicate one. Add disturbing intrusive thoughts to the mix that you have no control over, and no wonder many new mamas feel unsettled, especially in the early days. The tricky thing about our feelings is that whatever we feel is valid. If you feel sadness, you genuinely are sad. If you feel fear, you truly are frightened; however, just because your emotions are valid doesn't necessarily mean they're rational. Given that our thoughts activate corresponding emotions, an irrational thought will result in an irrational emotion. As new mothers, what we feel, especially toward our beloved baby, can be so profound that we often find ourselves spiraling with anxiety as we lose our grip from wellness. So, what to do when we get stuck in perturbing feelings of doom and gloom? It's our behaviors that make the difference.

Behaviors

Of the three very basic foundations to human functioning, our behavior is the only element that we have direct control over because it involves our conscious choice. Whether you choose to delight yourself with a plate of chocolate-covered strawberries is directly within your control. You might criticize yourself and feel guilt afterward, or be glad to have indulged. Nevertheless, the act of consuming what's in front of you is determined by your actions. Similarly, whether you purposefully think of the yellow duck or resist it is also directly within your control. One action will defuse the impact of the image while the other will draw more attention to it just by resisting it. Either way, how you respond to the intrusive yellow duck is completely up to you.

Albeit, we have no direct control over our thoughts or emotions, we do have direct control over how we respond to them. When an upsetting thought about baby interrupts and elicits anxious feelings, how we react to the thought will determine what happens next. For instance, if you have an intrusive thought of dropping your innocent newborn that naturally triggers perturbing feelings, you might respond by evading having to hold baby altogether. However, this avoidance behavior will likely disrupt your bond with baby. On the other hand, if your reaction to the thought is to ignore its silliness, then you will continue to hold and bond with your little one without missing a beat.

By making intentional choices, including our actions and reactions to intrusive thoughts and corresponding emotions, we exert direct control over our behaviors even when they're difficult or uncomfortable to make. Hence, whether holding your helpless infant with the possibility of dropping them is distressing or not, the choice to pick up your little one is still directly within your control. In essence, you have no direct control over your thoughts because of your continuous stream of sensory inputs, and you have no direct control over your emotions because they're triggered from thoughts. You do have direct control over your behaviors. When you put forth intentional actions that support your wellness with baby, the nature of your thoughts and resulting emotions will also gradually change since you'll no longer be giving unintended attention to your anxious monster.

Decoding the Biology of Anxiety That Maintains Intrusive Thoughts

Anxiety is a common feeling for many new and expectant mothers. Throughout pregnancy, childbirth, and the postpartum period, the level of uncertainty and new responsibilities all add to the experience of stress and anxious thoughts. If you have doubts about your ability to care for your newborn, know that your worry has been shared by many moms. Yet, despite the uncomfortable bodily sensations, anxiety is a necessary component to our survival. One that keeps us alert and prepared to respond to any perceived danger. As a new mom with the added burden to keep baby safe and protected, our antennae are naturally raised to detect any potential harm.

At the core of anxiety is your body's "fight-or-flight" response. Its job is to simply react to whatever you perceive as harmful. Like the classic caveman example, if you walk out of your cave and see a large saber-toothed tiger, your natural instinct is to protect yourself and baby. To do this well, your body quickly becomes flooded with stress hormones. Adrenaline and cortisol propel your body to react so you can fight or flee from the danger-ous threat. For instance, your breathing intensifies, bringing oxygen to your lungs, while your heart beats rapidly to pump blood, carrying oxygen throughout your body. As your muscles tighten for fighting or fleeing, you may tremble, have chills, and be a sweaty mess. Depending on how long your fight-or-flight alarm remains activated, you could consequently have headaches or body aches from holding your muscles tightly. You may even experience diarrhea or constipation because energy is diverted to your limbs for a prolonged period, leaving minimal energy to your core for digestion. You might feel these bodily sensations as discomfort and inter-pret them as anxiety, except your body is only doing its job in the face of a perceived threat.

On the other hand, let's say you see a harmless kitty cat instead of a threatening tiger. In that case, your fight-or-flight alarm wouldn't be trig-gered all because you hadn't perceived potential harm. As a matter of fact, your body's alarm system is extremely compliant and responds to whatever you perceive. It can't tell the difference whether your interpretations are accurate or not and just oblige. If you interpret your situation as safe like the kitty cat, it follows your perception and remains immobilized. If you sense sabre-toothed danger and conjure up thoughts of impending danger, it obeys and quickly rallies up your stress hormones to activate your body into full defensive mode to protect you and baby.

Unfortunately, most of us dislike feeling anxious, and when we do, we attempt to avoid whatever triggered it. Here again, how we react to our thoughts of perceived danger and resulting emotional response is directly within our control. If you interpret a situation with terrorizing thoughts of the sabre-toothed tiger, then your fight-or-flight alarm will saturate your body with anxious feelings. In contrast, if you perceive the same situation with non-threatening thoughts of the kitty cat, then your body will not be inundated with stress hormones. The choice to react in one way or another is completely yours.

Nevertheless, when we react by avoiding the perceived threat, not only do we miss getting corrective feedback about its lack of danger, we also bestow more attention and power to the situation than what it may actu-ally deserve. Keep in mind, whatever we resist, persists. Thus, try to not think of the tiger, and it becomes larger. Try to not think about dropping baby, and the idea becomes more forceful. Now, instead, only think about *DROPPING BABY, DROPPING BABY, Dropping Baby, Dropping Baby, dropping baby, dropping baby, droppingbaby, droppingbaby, droppingbabydroppingbaby...* Will you feel anxious?

As a new mom with the weight of having to protect and care for a helpless infant, the thought of dropping your baby is naturally a daunting one. Though following the initial startle, how you respond to the thought will determine whether your anxiety monster evolves or retreats. If you recognize the thoughts as silly intrusive nonsense, then the initial distress will be more easily dismissed. Conversely, if you attribute frightening sabretoothed qualities to the thoughts, then your fight-or-flight alarm will initiate, leaving you with lasting feelings of dread. Alas, the more you react by avoiding the thought and feared situation, the louder it becomes. Alternatively, purposefully and repeatedly thinking of the unmentionable sabre-toothed tiger will paradoxically reduce its terrorizing influences.

Remember, you have no direct control over your thoughts or emotions, and only have direct control over your behaviors. How you respond and react to your thoughts impact whether your fight-or-flight alarm will activate a natural stress response in service of protecting your wellness with baby. When you resist avoidance and push through to confront what's feared, you're also empowering yourself to meet motherhood and life's challenges with courage, vigor, and tenacity. To remain confident and resilient throughout your motherhood journey, try to embrace versus avoid each trial and tribulation despite the dreaded thoughts and feelings.

Transforming Your Fight-or-Flight Anxiety into Productive Energy

When we think about the body's fight-or-flight response, it's usually associated with perceived threats that trigger our experience of anxiety like the classic caveman and sabre-toothed tiger analogy. Less often do we connect this physiological response to feelings of excitement or the productive use of energy. Nonetheless, our fight-or-flight response prepares our body to meet challenges whether the emotional valance of the situation is comprised of anxiety or excitement.

For instance, let's say you agree to go on a skydiving trip with a friend. Depending on your proclivity for extreme sports, you may anticipate jumping out of a plane with terror or exhilaration. Either way, your body experiences a similar, objective fight-or-flight biological response, most noted for its sudden adrenaline rush. Both you and your friend will feel rapid heart rates, heavy breathing, tense muscles, sweatiness, and shaky limbs. However, your mind interprets these biological events subjectively. Hence, while your friend might find the experience enthralling, you might think quite differently.

In fact, when we talk about anxiety, fear, or stress, we're communicating our subjective experience of our body's objective fight-or-flight arousal. This response plays a role in both anxiety and excitement depending on our interpretations. Public speaking can be perceived as an intimidatingly judgmental task or a rewarding social undertaking. Athletes can easily succumb to the pressures of competitive sports or utilize the added energy from their fight-or-flight adrenaline to defy the odds and defeat an opponent. Similarly, we can interpret the demands of new motherhood with trepidation, which will create a vicious feedback loop that reinforces the perception of anxiety. Or we can react to the challenges of motherhood as a stimulating opportunity to learn about baby and strengthen our valuable bond. Responding with this alternate perception helps to override feelings of fear and foster a positive feedback loop that reinforces the sense of productive energy.

As mothers, we invest our entire being to our children, often before they're born and, sometimes, before they're even conceived. Accordingly, the burden we carry to protect them, our investment, is immense, which naturally heightens our scrutiny for potential threats. Still, you can encourage a positive feedback loop by perceiving your body's fight-or-flight experience as motivating energy to securely bond with baby instead of avoidance reactions that will distance you from baby. When you interpret the fight-or-flight energy in this productive way instead of labeling it as uncomfortable warnings, then you'll be that much closer to adjusting the sabre-tooth for the kitty cat when you need to reclaim your wellness.

Avoiding Intrusive Thoughts Will Only Reinforce Them

Some mothers might say that they've never had to tolerate relentless anxiety at intense levels until their motherhood journey began. Others might say that their fears and worries quickly spiraled from manageable to unbearable at the blink of an eye since becoming a new mother. How do once benign thoughts become intrusively powerful so quickly? Why do we get so swiftly imprisoned by our fears? The yellow duck principle applies here—whatever we resist, persists.

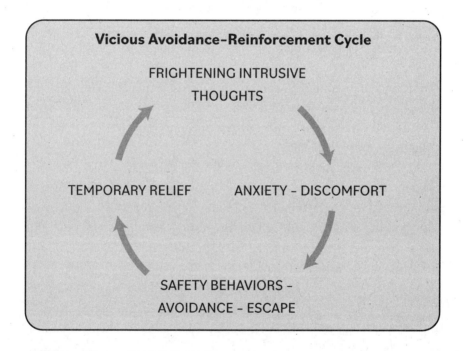

We all have intrusive thoughts—some more salient than others. Sometimes, the thoughts arise as images or sensations. Nevertheless, the ones that are more prominent tend to create the most uncomfortable feelings like anxiety, guilt, devastation, or horror, just to name a few. These distressing emotions are induced because we actively deem the thoughts as forbidden. We might wonder why we have such awful thoughts. We might try to reason where these unintentional sensations come from. We might even judge ourselves for allowing such appalling images into our minds. Just by attempting to answer such questions in order to expunge our moral involvement, we consequently end up taking more ownership for having such involuntary thoughts. By asking *why, how, where,* and *what if* questions, we inherently bestow more power and credence to the initial thought, image, or sensation, all resulting in anxiety and discomfort.

Since no one wants to feel uncomfortable, and we are a society that prioritizes happiness with little tolerance for discomfort, what do you do to feel better when you have no direct control over intrusive thoughts or upsetting emotions? One option is to prevent the uncomfortable thoughts and feelings by engaging in safety behaviors to feel protected or by avoiding the situations linked to the thoughts altogether. Whether these behaviors seem rational or have a magical, superstitious quality to them, whenever they're put to practice, you achieve some initial relief. However, this relief is only temporary until the next revolting intrusive thought arises. In turn, you repeat this cycle again and again to achieve the much-desired relief because you cannot bear to tolerate the uncomfortable feelings stemming from the intrusive thoughts.

Alas, the next intrusive thought will most certainly surface since you have no direct control over the type of thoughts that enter and exit your awareness based on the billions of stimuli you perceive. Moreover, distressing thoughts will naturally trigger distressing emotions. However, this doesn't mean that you have to be stuck in this vicious anxiety cycle, perpetuating the same loop to reach reprieve. Remember, how you respond to those initial thoughts and subsequent emotions will determine how powerful the thoughts become. Fortunately, there are other ways to react to intrusive thoughts rather than relying on magical safety schemes that only deliver short-term relief.

In fact, the temporary relief you gain from staying on the rat wheel, albeit potent, is one of the anxiety monster's most reliable tricks. That sigh of relief is a persuasive reinforcer of all things that cause you distress. As a new sleep-deprived mom, what you lack most is reprieve. Hence, it's easy to repeat the behaviors that seem to give you the temporary relief you crave. In turn, however, you'll unintentionally become a mindless puppet without cognizance of the strings being pulled to keep you going. In the long run, repeatedly performing excessive safety practices like a puppet in response to dreaded intrusive thoughts will be more energy-wasting than energy-preserving. Since the relief is only temporary, a more reasonable long-term solution is to do nothing and carry on because that's what you do have control over and intrusive thoughts, frankly, lack meaning. When you can acknowledge a frightening intrusive thought as just another thought, then it doesn't have impetus to activate the anxiety that urges you to behave in senseless puppet ways.

Let's understand this avoidance–reinforcement cycle with a more relatable analogy. We've all experienced headaches, some of which are mild while others have migraine qualities. For those of us who are less tolerant, we might anticipate the first intrusive sensations of an impending headache with unease that prompt us to take precautionary action. This safety measure might consist of taking an over-the-counter medication like ibuprofen, taking deep breaths to induce more oxygen into the brain, or even taking a nap to rest our head. Any number of these protocols may or may not work for you. Nevertheless, say your headache reliever of choice is to take ibuprofen, and within the hour of consuming it, your dreaded headache dissipates as you gain reprieve. However, headaches come and go, and often occur spontaneously. When the next tension headache approaches and you're once again feeling apprehensive, what will you do?

Likely, you will take another ibuprofen at the first sensation of an intrusive headache—because it worked. Though, let's say you're out of this magical pill and resort to taking deep breaths instead. While breathing in oxygen helped to reduce inflammation, this approach took over an hour as you endured the agony rather than getting a quick escape. As you reflect on that terrible experience, you immediately replace the empty bottle of magical ibuprofen to avoid having to tolerate another such episode without protection. Thus, when the next intrusive headache arises, what will you do? Most likely, you'd take the magical ibuprofen again because it worked, even though this escape method will need to be repeated for future intrusive headaches.

Simply stated, we are driven to avoid discomfort and feel relief. Whatever we do that delivers quick relief, rational or irrational, is reinforced to be repeated. When a new mama has dreaded intrusive thoughts of potential harm to her baby, the ensuing emotions are often felt profoundly. Yet again, how you react to the frightening thoughts will either warrant meaning to the thoughts or not. One response will imprison you to a perpetual state of puppetry. To reclaim wellness for both you and baby, the more empowering response is to do nothing and carry on—because whatever you resist, persists.

Ruminado: The Domino Effect of Worries and Negative Thinking

We've all had the experience of lying awake at night, waiting to fall into deep sleep only to be distracted by one worrisome thought after another. For instance, you remember that you'd forgotten to put baby's laundry into the dryer and turn on the bottle sterilizer for the next feeding. As you imagine the wet bottles sitting in the closed storage container, your mind starts to wander to what-if-land. "What if there's not enough air circulating in the sterilizer container?" "What if the bottles have already sat in there for too long?" "What if the moisture gets trapped inside the bottles and starts to grow tiny mold spores?" "What if I can't see the mold and wouldn't know it's still there after cleaning the bottles again?" "What if baby gets sick from drinking mold, or worst, gets some unknown long-term illness?"

Just as you start to go down the rabbit hole of all things germy and moldy, another unfinished business interrupts your worried mind. You're out of baby butt cream and remember noticing the early symptoms of a looming diaper rash on your little one tonight. As you make a mental note to pick some up in the morning, a disturbing intrusive image of inflamed skin on baby's buttocks assaults your thoughts. Once again, you drift farther into what-if-land as opposed to dreamland, unintentionally awakening your worried mind further. "What if the store is out of butt cream?" "What if the rash gets worse by morning?" "What if baby's bum ends up full of painful sores?" Lying there still, the wave of each troublesome thought inherently sparks the next, just like the chain reaction of a carefully lined domino set.

Unfortunately, worrisome thoughts are most disruptive when it's least convenient—either when we are underwhelmed or overwhelmed. When our minds are quiet and underwhelmed, our brains slow down with fewer stimuli to keep them occupied. Needing less cognitive effort during calm states allows more mental space for thoughts to naturally enter and exit our awareness. Because we are instinctively attuned to our thoughts and emotions when we have the mental bandwidth, we simply become more aware of worries and anxieties. At the forefront of our concerns is the responsibility to nurture and protect our treasured baby—the emotional investment we've devoted ourselves to. As such, when it's quiet, when we try to rest our fatigued mind and body, our brain naturally drifts to intrusive thoughts and worries about our little one.

On the other end of the spectrum, when our minds are overwhelmed with insufficient mental space to adequately attend to mom life demands, our fight-or-flight energy kicks in to assist us. As stress hormones inundate our body into action, our brain is quickly prompted to be vigilant for all potential threats to our well-being and all unfinished tasks still on our shoulders. However, with limited mental bandwidth to discern whether a stressor is trivial or substantial, and the proclivity as a new mom to deem situations as harmful, our minds are more naturally attuned to negative thinking while our body is already distressed. This cycle that alternates between periods of mostly overwhelm and brief interludes of underwhelm during new motherhood provides a convenient opportunity for our anxiety monster to harass us with unwelcomed thoughts and worries contributing to our unwellness.

Nonetheless, when the worry train is unleashed, it has a domino effect. Each negative thought that is triggered becomes more likely to elicit other negative thoughts. Like a tornado that picks up speed and strength, the more energy we feed to the string of worries, the faster it will spiral into a frenzy of ruminating negative thoughts. Moreover, when the worry train is loose, we resort to ruminating as our misguided attempt at problem-solving for a future-oriented dilemma—baby's diaper rash, for instance. We get stuck analyzing solutions to anticipated problems because the repetitive thinking *feels* constructive and useful in the moment; however, it actually creates a vicious feedback loop. Just like the avoidance–reinforcement cycle, ruminating over potentially distressing events and their possible solutions might generate some reprieve in the moment, but it's at the expense of your long-term motherly sanity, with no single solution guaranteed.

This is why the what-if-land of mom life is so attractive. The exact purpose of *what if* questions is to anticipate possible catastrophic consequences while contemplating various solutions. As a new mom with the responsibility to protect and nurture baby, we are innately tasked with the duty to anticipate potential harm to our helpless little one. However, when our brain is stuck in a "ruminado," trying to escape in order to explore realistic solutions or optimistic outcomes gets even more challenging. Hence, the domino effect is maintained. By replaying the unhelpful worries over and over again, we unintentionally and implicitly hold the worry train in very high regards. Very quickly, your mind spirals faster and faster with other worrisome thoughts about baby, each consuming more energy, leaving you with brain fog and fatigue until you're completely drained. Therefore, not only is this approach to maintaining your maternal wellness impractical, it essentially attaches more value to the worry itself than what you intended.

As a matter of fact, in what-if-land, a ruminado will overpower any rational thinking and annihilate effective decision making. Only when it's interrupted by other mom life demands or when your supply of energy is completely drained, leaving you in a state of burnout, will it weaken and dissipate. Whether this ruminado dies a quick death or a slow one is entirely up to you. How you react to an intrusive thought of your precious baby will determine the weight it carries and how long the experience will last. The more you imbue intrusive thoughts and worries with meaning and value, the more energy they gain. Conversely, when you don't attribute significance to senseless worries, they rapidly loses their forcefulness. One consumes the mental bandwidth that a new mama lacks, while the other saves it for the real sabre-toothed threat.

Changing Behaviors to Change Thoughts and Emotions

Can old habits be reshaped to honor your maternal wellness? According to the science of neuroplasticity, they can indeed. As you're now aware, behaviors, thoughts, and emotions are all interconnected and influence each other in a cyclical way. While you may not have direct control over the presence of anxious thoughts and worries, you do have control over how they affect your mother-child attachment. As a new mama, changing what you do and how you react to frightening intrusive thoughts will determine the subsequent thoughts and emotions and influence your connection with precious baby. If you want to keep the ruminado from dominating, you'll have to break vicious anxiety cycles and untenable old habits.

The good news is that our brain is neuroplastic and has the ability to change and adapt in response to our experiences to create new healthy habits. Change how you respond to whatever frightens you and a new mental network of healthier habits becomes established. On the other hand, continue old habits that rob you of your motherly wellness and you'll remain in the same stuck mindset. Whichever path is repeatedly reinforced is the one that gets sturdier. One will foster an authentic bond with baby without the sabre-tooth's undue influence, while the other will undoubtedly energize your relationship with the anxiety monster.

Ultimately, our brain has an incredible capacity to learn, change, and adapt throughout our lives if we're intentional about it. Since what you do determines how you feel and subsequent thoughts you have, intentionally changing how you respond to intrusive frightening thoughts is the first step to form new productive memories and healthy neural pathways. Thus, instead of reacting to elusive dreaded thoughts with avoidance, unwarranted safety protocols, or being stuck in a ruminado, a new mama needs more efficient methods.

The next part of this book will give you practical solutions to get out of your head. Each section comes with specific skills for practice that are broken down into achievable steps as I share my experience helping Remi, Kendall, Madelyn, and Wilmina reclaim their wellness on their motherhood journey. By practicing these evidence-based strategies that support your sanity being a new mom, your uncomfortable thoughts and emotions will organically become gentler as healthier neural connectivity gets established. Now, let's begin Part II to practice the habits that will nurture your bond with baby so you too can reclaim your wellness on your motherhood journey.

PRACTICAL SOLUTIONS TO GET OUT OF YOUR HEAD

Chapter 3

Expanding Comfort Through Discomfort

I once opened a fortune cookie with the message, "The best way to expand your comfort is through discomfort." Reflecting on this message as a new mom can be hard to fathom. How can I possibly experience any more discomfort than what I'm already going through? I'm sleep-deprived. I'm fatigued all the time. My body aches all over and is not in adequate shape. I don't have the support I need from my partner or family. My brain is foggy and I can't remember anything. I'm an emotional wreck. And I don't even know what I'm doing to be the best mom for my baby.

If this sounds familiar, you're not alone. Any new mom will agree that motherhood is the single hardest and oftentimes most thankless job that exists. The job description can involve anything and everything without a specific instruction manual that fits every parenting situation, leaving much to uncertainty. And that's where our fears, worries, and anxiety thrive—on doubt and uncertainty. Without a handbook to navigate through all the quandaries of parenting, no wonder our minds are often filled with "what if" ruminations and catastrophic frightening thoughts.

Does this mean you have to be stuck with Negative Nancy throughout your entire motherhood journey? Absolutely not! You don't have to let that anxious shadow overpower the precious bond with your baby or your maternal wellness. Motherhood can be one of the most rewarding, heartfelt, and joyous experiences. The trick is learning where your anxiety monster lurks and equipping yourself with knowledge and proven strategies to tackle it.

The Paradox of Uncertainty

According to Benjamin Franklin, the only certainties in life are death and taxes. This means everything else is left to chance. Whether you're wondering about your financial stability, job security, your health and that of your family, or even the safety of your child, the truth is it's all indefinite from moment to moment. Sure, you may have some awareness of this current moment with a bit of certainty. You may know with absolute certainty that you're breathing right now, and everything that you can see or touch exists; however, you're never really guaranteed certainty in the next moment or even within this moment...except for death and taxes. How can that be? Try this with me.

I want you to imagine a loved one. Get a steady picture of this person in your mind whether it's your partner, a parent, a sibling, or even your innocent child. Can you see their smile? Can you feel their joy? If this person is not currently with you, what do you see them doing right now? Do they feel real in your imagination? Are they currently safe—right this moment? How do you know for sure? As difficult as it is to imagine harm occurring to those we love, the truth is you never know. Unless you're currently with your loved one or connected with them on a digital device, you actually don't know for certain of their well-being. Yet every day, we go through life believing those whom we love are okay. You simply trust the unknown and tolerate the uncertainties all around, whether consciously or not.

That's the paradox. The only thing we know for sure is that most everything in life is uncertain. This loophole is where our anxiety monster lurks: within the vast shadow of not knowing. For a new mother, this shadow can encompass endlessly frightening possibilities because pregnancy and the newborn stage are when our baby is most fragile. Our innocent infants are truly helpless and cannot live on their own. They need us to ensure their safety, well-being, and health. They rely on our ability to care for their every whim and need not just to survive but also to thrive. That is a heavy weight of responsibility for a new mom, especially in the early days and months when sleep and energy are often depleted.

Worrying Isn't the Answer

The influence of uncertainty is especially powerful in the early days of motherhood—whether you have just conceived, are in your third trimester and about to deliver, or you're getting acquainted with your newborn in the fourth trimester. Truth is, anxiety and fear thrive on doubt. When the stakes are high, our mind tends to spiral the fastest to the worst possible thoughts and worries.

If you're a new mom, you just might have endless worries of how to keep your helpless newborn from any possible harm. You might be questioning whether you've accidentally contaminated their milk with toxins from inadequate cleaning of bottles. You might even believe that you've consumed harmful foods that baby is now ingesting through breastmilk. You might have intrusive thoughts of accidentally dropping your baby, carelessly drowning baby in the bath, falling asleep on baby, resulting in sudden infant death syndrome (SIDS), or countless other fears.

You have these frightening thoughts because you care deeply, and in your desire to protect your helpless infant, worrying is the misguided attempt to keep them from harm. Except, as you've already learned, constantly worrying about potential threats and ruminating about exit strategies or safety protocols only take your mental and emotional bandwidth away from this cherished time with baby, resulting in your unwellness.

In fact, whenever you're caught in a frenzy of anxiety, your mind gets stuck either in the past, haunted by daunting memories, or travels to distant futures to prevent any catastrophic possibilities. On the other hand, there is no room in the present moment for anxious thoughts. When you are simply *being* in the present, your mind isn't able to sneak away to the endless images of potential harm to baby. Instead, you're able to connect, gaze, and adore their lovable sweetness while forming the strong attachment needed for their well-being. If you want to ensure the health of your child, spending invaluable time worrying isn't the answer. Instead, taking time to secure your mother-infant bond is the better choice. To do this, you'll have to dismiss your worries while tolerating the uncomfortable uncertainties that naturally come with life.

> ### Time to Flex Your Mental Muscles
>
> Now that you understand why avoidance of feared intrusive thoughts and worries only strengthen their power, let's take a look at some specific strategies to embrace uncertainty and truly expand your comfort together with baby.

Making Room for Uncertainty

Uncertainty will certainly bring discomfort. That's exactly where your anxious monster thrives—in that uncomfortable space of not knowing for sure. Your need to know with conviction—that baby is safe and that you're not a terrible mother—is how your anxious mind gets trapped in spiraling circles. As absurd as it is to believe in the absolute certainty of anything other than death and taxes, many mamas still try hard to seek this meaningless illusion that only triggers further worry and dread. To tolerate the discomfort of not always knowing everything means that we have to make room for uncertainty because that unquestionable reality is the essence of living where authentic bonding with baby occurs.

I know it's easier said than done. We are creatures of comfort and one essential factor that provides comfort is knowing with absolute certainty that our children are healthy, safe, and happy. That's why we drive our minds to insanity with worries and dreadful intrusive thoughts. However, since it's not realistic to have assurance with absolute certainty that our loved ones will always be free from harm, we have to accept the uncertainties of their lives and adapt to being tolerant with the unknown. The truth is, unless you have a magical crystal ball or voodoo abilities to see into the future, you have to embrace the reality that not much is certain and most anything is possible.

Making room for uncertainty means actively recognizing that life is often ambiguous and unpredictable. As uncomfortable as it is to fathom all of the possible dangers that exist in life, uncertainty is a natural and inevitable reality. Intentionally acknowledging this is what will allow you to tolerate uncertainty without becoming overwhelmed or paralyzed when you feel the dark shadows of not knowing enveloping your mind. In all honesty, you already accept some degree of uncertainty every day. Whenever you leave your house, how do you know for sure that you'll return? Yet, you leave anyway. Whenever you step away from baby, how do you know for certain that you'll reconnect? Nonetheless, you do it anyway even with hesitation. Taking this blind leap despite not knowing what will happen next is the embodiment of living an authentic life—one that will nurture your bond with baby.

To expand your comfort zone by making room for uncertainty, incorporate these guidelines into your everyday living:

1. Whenever you find yourself spending excessive time ruminating, researching, or asking the same questions in a bazillion different ways to be absolutely sure, cultivate the momentum to sit with the anxiety and discomfort that come with uncertainty without attempting to control it. Watch out for unhealthy reactions to uncertainty, such as needless worrying, intentional avoidance, or mindlessly seeking reassurance that only creates space for further doubt.

2. Test out your beliefs that you must know with absolute certainty by challenging your prediction that not knowing is disastrous. The next time you feel the urge to seek reassurance when a doubt arises, identify the catastrophic consequence and resist the urge to determine the actual outcome. Use these experiments to replace the irrational need for certainty with more realistic tolerance for uncertainty.

3. Embrace uncertainty as an opportunity to become stronger mentally and emotionally. Not knowing provides the space for learning, discovery, and growth. Exploring new possibilities from the

unexpected is what fuels excitement, fresh experiences, and meaning in life. Imagine how rudimentary and monotonous life would be if everything was the same and predictable day in and day out.

4. When you're stuck in unhelpful ruminations to ascertain answers that have no specific outcomes, shift your focus to what is within your control. Fixating on what is beyond your control will only keep the vicious loop of uncertainty spiraling. By actively tolerating the unknown and accepting this reality, you're expanding the comfort zone that will ultimately strengthen your bond with baby.

Kendall's Experience

When Kendall first sat with me, she was still grieving over the loss of her two previous pregnancies—both of which occurred in the second trimester. Although the miscarriages were caused by chromosomal abnormalities beyond her control, she still wrestled with feelings of guilt and shame that kept her from sharing her grief with family and friends, including her husband. Instead, Kendall remained emotionally isolated while she silently feared the possibility of losing her current baby. In fact, our first session was the very first time Kendall allowed herself to talk about her anguish. Nevertheless, the weight and responsibility of maintaining this third pregnancy now fueled terrifying intrusive thoughts that she will miscarry once again along with the emotional aftermath that will follow. At every prenatal appointment, Kendall hoped to be reassured by the OB that her baby was safe, except she was instead reminded of her baby's fragility from the excessive warnings she received.

In our sessions, Kendall was assured that her apprehensive worries were valid and understandable given the very real heartaches she endured. Nevertheless, her dreaded intrusive thoughts of suffering another miscarriage weren't only unhelpful, they also limited her recognition that this catastrophic outcome wasn't the only possibility. To be well, Kendall was encouraged to make room for uncertainty along with all of life's possibilities because that's the nature of real living. In place of avoiding past hurts, we made space to process the painful thoughts and emotions while embracing her strength in doing so. We practiced sitting with the discomfort of not knowing the actual outcome of this pregnancy, rather than creating an alleged narrative filled with false assumptions and predictions. Most importantly, to maintain calm, Kendall learned to shift her focus to what was within her control—acknowledging all the things that were going well with her pregnancy. For Kendall, not knowing with 100 percent certainty whether she would carry her pregnancy to term wasn't the problem; spending hours ruminating over this uncertainty was what boosted her anxiety monster's strength.

Making room for uncertainty allows you to adapt to an attitude that coexists with not knowing what the future holds and accepting the unpredictability of life. This process isn't easy and will be really uncomfortable at first, just like any training we commit to. As painful as it may be to allow terrifying images and catastrophic consequences into our minds, that's the only way to accept reality. Once you're able to tolerate the actuality of uncertainty, then your anxious shadow won't have the opportunity to play tricks and your mind will be freer to bond genuinely with baby. All of which will only enhance your and baby's resilience in time.

Flexibility in EVERYTHING

Whatever you resist, persists. Remember that yellow duck? Whenever you try to *not* think of something or attempt to avoid those frightening intrusive thoughts, you're actually dedicating more energy to the taboo image and terrifying thought. Naturally, when we worry about all the ways our baby may be harmed, our minds travel to the worst possibilities with the associated horrifying images. Depending on how we interpret the daunting thoughts and images, we may conclude that our baby is not safe, that we're not doing enough to keep baby healthy, that we're not good enough parents, or that there's something wrong with us for even having such terrifying thoughts. Our instinct is to stop the thoughts in their tracks to keep them from spiraling, except this misguided attempt only directs extra attention and energy to the unwanted images. As a result, we end up with a flurry of more intrusive frightening thoughts and feelings of dread, anxiety, and guilt. Try as you may to stop the ruminado, each attempt will only leave you more overwhelmed, physically exhausted, mentally fatigued, and emotionally drained.

To escape this end, the better choice is to take the paradoxical approach and embrace flexibility. How? Let's first define it. Flexibility is the ability to bend without breaking in order to adjust and adapt. This quality, whether applied physically or mentally, is crucial to resiliency. When we practice a flexible mindset, we're *making* room for infinite possibilities along a continuum and not just spiraling to the worst outcomes and explanations. This means shifting your thinking from avoidance of those horrifying images of harm or believing you must be ill-equipped to parent, to being open to the various uncertainties that come with life—both positive and negative.

Unlike disturbing images of harm to baby, a simple fleeting thought doesn't have the weight to agonize you because it doesn't come attached with negative associations. When you're caught off guard by intrusive thoughts, your mind gets stuck on the vivid details of the feared images and worries. Whether you fear your baby choking, drowning, suffocating, or being physically injured in some other way, intrusive thoughts only hold value if you let them. With the overwhelming responsibility to keep our helpless infant healthy and safe, especially in those early days and months, our brains are constantly scanning the environment and purposefully looking for ways that baby might be harmed. Thus, the problem isn't in the thoughts themselves but, rather, in how we interpret the thoughts.

Mental flexibility helps us think outside the box and find different ways to interpret those thoughts, disturbing as they may be. It moves us from feeling defined by having such horrific thoughts to appreciating their adaptive purpose that keeps us vigilant on our baby's safety. It creates distance between those unhelpful worries of harm to baby and our consequential emotions of fear, shame, helplessness, or incompetence. It makes room for all the uncertain possibilities that can affect baby while honoring our own essence to mother the tiny bundle of responsibility. When we no longer perceive these intrusive thoughts with negative judgment, we're mentally changing the direction of the rigid thoughts and detaching from the power they have on our beliefs and identity.

Garnering a flexible growth mindset will require self-awareness and intentional effort. Integrate these principles into your daily practice, and especially whenever you're stuck in a spiraling thought, to minimize its unwarranted impact:

1. The next time an intrusive atrocious thought surfaces, rather than resisting it, which only persists it, give your thoughts the permission and flexibility to flow through. Attend to the thoughts with a curious mind no matter how distressing they may be, in order to diminish their power. As you begin to break the anxious reactions formerly attached to the avoided thoughts, you'll gain space to discover new observations that might've been previously obscured.

2. Shift your mindset to other potential interpretations to deter your dreaded intrusive thoughts and worries from spiraling to their worst consequences. By considering alternative possibilities, you're cultivating flexibility in your thinking to develop a growth mindset. Having this ability to reflect from different viewpoints will also help you handle obstacles from a proactive problem-solving approach.

3. Approach rigid thoughts and challenging worries as opportunities for learning and growth instead of hurdles to be avoided. Embrace the adaptive purpose of these thoughts and apply your insights to future thoughts and worries. Bending this fixed mindset will reveal perspectives from various lenses and change the meaning previously attributed to the frightening thoughts.

4. Embrace flexibility and uncertainty as natural and real by asking yourself whether your beliefs from distressing intrusive thoughts are based on evidence and proof. Although negative assumptions from thoughts can *feel* real, they are not based in fact, and thus will only keep you in a rigid mindset that will continue to hold you back from building a resilient bond with baby.

Madelyn's Experience

Madelyn's doula suggested that she meet with me to help manage her prolonged baby blues. When she did finally reach out during the second month postpartum, she quickly shared about her persistent difficulty bonding with her baby that triggered a variety of unorthodox thoughts: Aside from feeling overwhelmed and fatigued, Madelyn also felt detached from her two-month-old boy and dreaded being alone with the responsibilities of her baby. Being a new single mom, she was far from feeling well or supported and felt constant guilt for wanting to relinquish her motherhood role. In fact, having such a challenging adjustment, Madelyn spent more time attempting to avoid the intrusive thoughts that bombarded her mind than connecting and getting acquainted with her little one. She simply relied on her doula to instruct her about her baby's needs and care without learning about him more directly. Madelyn felt terrible and regularly blamed herself for her seeming lack of effort and perceived failure.

After presenting her experiences to me, Madelyn learned that her symptoms consisted of more than just the baby blues and warranted diagnoses of postpartum anxiety and depression. She struggled with having to care for a newborn alone when even trying to tend to a baby's needs in a two-parent household was hard. To break free from intrusive thoughts that contributed to anxiety and depression, avoidance and blame wasn't the answer. Madelyn's first step was to build flexibility into her thoughts and consider alternative explanations to change the negative associated meanings that she had failed as a mother. Bending the rigid beliefs that her difficulty attaching with baby was her fault allowed her to accept the reality that postpartum anxiety and depression was the reason. In essence, Madelyn was embracing a growth mindset.

Eventually, she realized that she didn't abandon her baby as her anxious monster tricked her to believe. On the contrary, despite her brain fog and exhaustion, she persisted and found other ways to manage her motherly duties. She managed baby bottles, laundry, and general upkeep while her doula tended to direct baby demands. She stayed close and watched carefully as her doula handled her baby expertly. And she rested when baby slept. As the days and weeks unfolded, Madelyn continued to *adopt flexibility into her experiences by discovering other observations that challenged her beliefs of being an unfit mother. She was responding to her baby's smiles as well as his cries with nurturance instead of dread. She held him more intently and naturally became more attuned to his needs. Practicing this flexible mindset helped her to see other positives around her, which increased confidence in her mothering role. All of this gave her the motivation she needed to connect more intimately with her baby, further dismissing her groundless intrusive thoughts and worries of doubt and incompetence.*

Exercising these adaptive skills will keep the mind agile to be truly free from the anxiety monster. A rigid mind keeps us stuck in the vicious cycle of terrifying thoughts and anxious emotions, while a flexible mind opens the window of possibilities and resiliency. When we practice flexibility in our thinking, doing, and being, our feelings of dread and anxiety will also change in time.

Dedicated Worry Times

Have you ever worried productively? Although it sounds counterintuitive, setting aside dedicated times in your day focused solely on your worries actually reduces stress and anxiety throughout the day. Remember, when we attempt to avoid frightening intrusive thoughts about our loved ones, we're actually giving these unwanted worries more attention and energy. Instead, the more productive option is to make room for these worries during specified times of the day.

You might be wondering why any loving mother would want to dedicate valuable time that she doesn't even have for such disheartening thoughts. In truth, these daunting worries have already been relentlessly feeding on your mind without your permission. That's why you're here reading this. These irritating thoughts simply pop up and invade your senses at the most inopportune times. For instance, while preparing baby's bottle, an unexpected worry emerges that you've neglected to sanitize sufficiently, resulting in milk that may now be contaminated with toxins. When feeding your child, your mind gets attacked with "what if" warnings of potential choking accidents. During bath time, you get hijacked by a stream of horrid images of the helpless terror on your little one's face if their body sinks under water. At bedtime, another alarming concern of SIDS surfaces once again as you reluctantly visualize baby suffocating, leaving you heartbroken and unable to rest. Even when you're not directly with your baby, you're flooded with worries of their entire journey from infancy throughout childhood.

In essence, dealing with untamed worries is like being injected with an IV drip, delivering unwanted thoughts from the time you're awake until the moments before falling into dreamland. Yet, by allocating specific periods of the day for these spontaneous intrusive worries, you are taking proactive measures to confine them to structured times of your choosing.

To make the most of your dedicated worry times, put these principles into practice at least once daily and more often if needed:

1. Writing a worry statement translates repetitive mental ruminations into specific acknowledgments on paper. Each worry statement is concise, with a beginning and an end, and is direct and to the point without further forecast. On the other hand, mental ruminations are a collection of spiraling thoughts with each diving deeper to a worse outcome. Imagine the difference between a runaway train accelerating at unsafe speeds compared to a properly functioning train making methodical stops along the way. A worry time does not provide the opportunity to get lost in ruminations.

2. Write each of your worry statements on paper instead of typing them on a digital device. Information is processed more thoughtfully and thoroughly when we take the time to actually write. Although typing is faster, the goal of this exercise is to introspectively and deliberately make room for unwanted worries and build your awareness of their excessive nature.

3. Schedule fifteen-minute periods using a timer. If the timer goes off before you've completed all of your worries, finish the last statement and put your pen down. By doing this, you're practicing delaying worries to the next scheduled period and containing that

IV drip to your selected time. Conversely, if you run out of worries before the timer goes off, then recycle worries you've already entertained. The pen or pencil doesn't stop writing for the full fifteen minutes. This will require discipline for some.

4. Choose a time during the day with the least likelihood of interruptions. Perhaps, it's after putting your baby down to sleep, or when a family member can take over childcare. It's preferable to schedule at least two worry times daily—one in the late morning and one in the late afternoon or early evening. If you can only dedicate one fifteen-minute period per day, then pick a time later in the day or early evening when you've built up and delayed enough worries for this task.

My Experience

I didn't meet Tristan for at least twelve hours after he was separated from my womb. When we arrived at Tristan's incubator in the NICU, tears quickly welled up in my eyes with perplexing emotions. On the one hand, I was thankful to finally meet my son. Yet, seeing him in the clear plastic box with feeding and breathing tubes taped to his mouth and nostrils triggered my worried mind to spiral. I was swiftly flooded with another storm of terrifying images and catastrophic possibilities. As I held Tristan close and gazed down at his porcelain skin, examining his eyes, nose, lips, ears, and all ten fingers and toes, my mind once again raced in full-blown circles with endless "what if" ruminations. My anxious worry monster peaked its ominous head and haunted me with ghastly thoughts of losing this precious love in my arms. What if something else happens, something worse? What if the respiratory distress caused damage to other organs? What if he dies? What if this was the only time I would ever have with him? The limited time I was granted to be with him now felt like a looming threat.

After thirty minutes or so, it was time for us to return to the maternity ward. Dash also needed me, and it was almost nursing time again. I watched the nurse take Tristan from my arms, gently placing him back into the incubator, all while the same lingering "what if" worries spiraled around my head like a stormy tornado. As we blew goodbye kisses to our son through the clear plastic box and my husband began wheeling me back to my room, I knew the intrusive images of doom wouldn't simply go away on their own. Rather than giving the worries free rein to terrorize me at their convenience, I recognized the need to take control and confine them to the dedicated times of my choosing. Despite being emotionally drained and physically exhausted, I took out my journal and pen after nursing Dash, turned on my cell phone timer, and began spelling out each worry that flooded my thoughts for the next fifteen minutes.

- *I'm worried I won't ever see my sweet boy again.*

- *I'm worried something else will hurt him.*

- *I'm worried the lack of oxygen has damaged his organs.*

- *I'm worried he won't have a fulfilling life.*

- *I'm worried he will live a hard life full of obstacles.*

- *I'm worried he will never recognize me.*

- *I'm worried that one day, I won't be here to protect him and provide for him.*

- *I'm worried we will never have the mother-child experiences I've always dreamed of.*

- *I'm worried Dash will never get to meet his twin brother.*

- *I'm worried Dash won't remember Tristan.*

- *I'm worried I won't remember Tristan.*

- *I'm worried I will forget this feeling of love for my boy.*

- *I'm worried Tristan will be forgotten.*

- *If I lose Tristan, I worry I won't be able to give Dash my full self.*

- *I'm worried Dash will resent me for not being fully available for him.*

- *I'm worried... I'm worried... I'm worried I won't be the mom for either of my boys I had always envisioned.*

- *I'm worried I will lose Tristan.*

- *I'm worried I may also lose Dash.*

- *I'm worried about losing this miraculous reality with my two precious loves.*

- *I'm worried my worrying will distract me from authentically connecting with my babies.*

- *I'm worried I've already ruined my bond with them and their attachment with me.*

- *I'm worried about losing Tristan.*

- *I'm worried about losing Dash.*

- *I'm worried about losing my boys.*

- *I'm worried this will be the last time I get to hold him in my arms.*

If you feel this task is tedious, I can certainly relate. Any routine can be tedious initially until it becomes an innate habit. Think of this as time dedicated to exercising your brain muscles and strengthening their elasticity to mentally free your mind from those frightening thoughts. With practice, you'll get the hang of it and will be more in charge of regulating those pesky intrusive worries. Unless you've already got a dedicated worry time scheduled, whenever you find yourself ruminating over worries like a runaway train or spiraling with dreaded intrusive thoughts, then it's time to take out a pen and paper to reclaim your wellness from your anxious monster.

Chapter 4

Doing the Hard Work of the Unthinkable

When was the last time you had an intrusive, frightening thought? Was it last night when you bathed baby? Maybe it occurred this morning when you fed baby? Or perhaps it's happening in this very moment being away from baby? As you've already learned, there's no controlling intrusive thoughts. Our anxiety monster has a mischievous way of provoking us with these unthinkable thoughts when it's least convenient. Some intrusive thoughts might be daunting and grotesque while others might be embarrassing and shameful. Nevertheless, being a new mama means it's rarely convenient for much of anything, never mind irritating intrusive thoughts.

Although, keep in mind that we all have intrusive thoughts. Let me repeat: **WE ALL HAVE INTRUSIVE THOUGHTS.** The ones you have are no more dangerous or alarming than anyone else's. If they were, then they wouldn't be considered "intrusive" and unwanted. While yours might be about baby drowning in the tub, your neighbor's might be about their cat falling into the toilet. What makes yours more powerful to you and your neighbor's more powerful to them isn't because either is more threatening. Rather, you simply care more deeply about your baby while your neighbor cares more deeply about their cat. So, your motherly love and protective nature easily render your intrusive thoughts as unthinkable, unacceptable, and intolerable because *you* care. Regardless of the nature of the thoughts, when they are intrusive, you know by now that avoiding them will have a paradoxical effect that only empowers them. Therefore, to reclaim your maternal wellness, we have to embrace the opposite and do the hard work of facing them.

Thinking of the Unthinkable

Sometimes, our pesky anxiety monster gets overly powerful. It vigorously claws into every beautiful thought and sensation, distorting them into horrid images, helpless fear, and appalling guilt. When we're feeling less resilient in these moments, the urge to run and hide from terrorizing intrusive thoughts can become irresistible and we simply give in. Though it may *feel* easier to escape and avoid our fears in the short run, we're all too aware by now that the momentary relief is fleeting before the next lightning bolt of frightening images returns.

When your reserves are depleted and daunting intrusive thoughts dominate, these tend to be the hardest moments to confront the unthinkable worries and images. Nevertheless, if you want to protect your bond with your baby, avoiding this hard work won't be helpful. To kick your cruel anxiety monster to the curb for the long run, you'll still have to find the strength to think of the unthinkable. Being prepared to fight back also means you'll have to practice for these difficult moments during the little time you have between feedings, diaper changes, cleaning, bathing baby— and, sometimes, ourselves if we're lucky to have that extra minute or two.

Like dedicated worry times, exposures involve thinking and doing the unthinkable, only with more intentional details. This is another exercise to strengthen our brain muscles that will become habit with repeated practice. Many may be wondering why any new mother would want to spend the little free time she has purposefully imagining details of harm to her helpless baby or to anyone? The answer is still the same: to attain an authentic bond with your sweet little one that is free from debilitating anxiety. Hence, rather than avoiding and losing ourselves to our unbearable fears for only temporary reprieve, confronting them through exposures over time will decrease the frequency and intensity of those struggling moments.

If you've never heard of exposure work, it's essentially a structured method to confront whatever troubles you, whether it be intrusive frightening images or having the courage to give a public speech. There are a number of benefits when we confront the unthinkable. For one, we begin to build tolerance to the triggers (people, places, objects, situations) of our discomfort the more we expose ourselves to them. When we avoid these triggers, we denote credence to the fears and bestow them with unnecessary power. On the other hand, when we confront the triggers, we're giving ourselves the opportunity to correct untested beliefs and arrive at more realistic conclusions about our worries. As exposures are practiced and repeated, we're also gaining confidence about our own capacity to manage the harassing intrusive thoughts while reclaiming the power from the anxiety prankster. Little by little, the intensity of our anxiety, shame, or guilt will decrease while the frequency of our intrusive thoughts, fears, or worries declines. To practice exposures, we must first gather information about our intrusive thoughts and our reactions to them.

Time to Flex Your Mental Muscles

Facing the unthinkable instead of avoiding intrusive thoughts is the only way to neutralize their torturing effects. These next strategies will give you the precise means and guidance to doing and thinking the hard work that will keep you healthily bonded with baby.

Identifying Anxious Rules to Normalize Doing What's Natural

When instigated, our natural mama bear response is to fiercely protect our loved ones from any potential threat, even when the threat is our own thoughts. We initially do this by trying to mentally block and escape the terrorizing images to avoid their stings. Later, our attempts might evolve to reasoning and rationalizing with ourselves or others to seek reassurance from our irrational worries. As the intrusive thoughts become more prevalent and persistent, we develop other creative ways to lessen their grip. Over time, as one deviceful method evolves into another, rules begin to generate in further mama bear attempts to assure baby's wellness from the unthinkable.

Maybe you've only made important decisions related to your fertility plans on days with "good" numbers. Or you've tried to force only pleasant thoughts when doing anything related to baby to magically ensure an optimal outcome. Perhaps you've attempted to cover up baby's bottoms during every diaper change to keep sinful genitalia thoughts out of your vision. Or you've attempted to avoid your baby altogether to maintain their safety from your possible negligence.

As you've learned from the vicious anxiety cycle from chapter 2, although these clever attempts initially help to keep the intrusive thoughts at bay, they quickly turn into rigid rules with each repetition. Without you even knowing, these rules of what you can and cannot do rob you of the costly bond with baby despite your longing to hold, caress, and be with your precious love. Since no rule demanded by your anxiety monster is practical or natural, you have to identify and break them one by one to regain your wellness and authentic connection with baby.

Figuring out the rules you feel compelled to follow means getting to know your anxiety monster well. Two mamas with contamination worries can have completely different experiences. One may obsess over toxic foods and environments during pregnancy that can harm her unborn baby, then meticulously inspect every source of chemical elements in ingredients and her surroundings. Another may attempt to prevent poisoning baby with potentially contaminated breast milk by switching to formula altogether. Identifying these specific rules will determine the precise content for the next steps in expanding your comfort through discomfort.

Having this knowledge will facilitate your ability to curb your anxious shadow more successfully. Remember, your anxiety monster is a task master who excessively warns you of the potential dangers and threats in your environment. Its goal is to simply scare and bully you into following its rules. It tricks you into thinking that you must protect your baby by complying with the rigid research and inspection of every possible toxin around you at the expense of your much-needed sleep. Or it spins you into a complete 180, deceiving you into believing that your own organic liquid gold is always poisoned from the potential toxins ingested from your foods, so man-made formula might somehow be better. Every time you obey, you gain a little bit of temporary relief, except you must obey the rules over and over again like a mindless robot.

To help you break free from this vicious chain and identify these meaningless rules, follow these guidelines. In doing so, imagine being an anxiety detective who investigates and uncovers all the ways your anxiety monster actually harms you and your baby in the guise of misguided help.

1. With a paper or digital notepad, identify specific triggers that cause you to feel anxious, frightened, guilty, disgusted, sad, worried, on edge, or any discomforting emotion. Triggers can be specific events like bathing and feeding, places like baby's crib and the laundry room, people like strangers and baby, or objects like bottles and car seats. Don't worry if you're unsure whether a trigger is related to your anxiety monster. We're just collecting as much data as available and can test them out later for clarity.

2. Along with the triggers, try to recognize and record the associated intrusive thoughts that are so terrifying. They may involve simple "if... then..." statements, or "I must... to prevent..." beliefs such as, "I must clean and sanitize each bottle seven times in this specific order to prevent any toxic chemical from lingering inside." They may also come to you as horrid images of harm and danger to your baby, such as imagining your helpless little one in the emergency department with tubes wrapped throughout their tiny body as a result of poisoning from your breastmilk.

3. Intrusive images and thoughts can be so alarming that they elicit strong urges to do something about the potentially catastrophic situation and prevent any possibility of harm. Thus, what does your anxiety monster have you doing to feel better and gain relief

for the threat to be less imminent? Determine all of the steps, sequence, and guidelines involved in your behaviors. These can be physical fixes, such as handwashing each bottle with seven pumps of organic detergent before scrubbing it for seven minutes with a dish brush followed by rinsing seven times under very hot water and finally placing them in the sanitizer for sixty minutes. These rules can also be mental solutions, such as visualizing without interruption your baby joyously playing in their playpen while giving them their formula whenever it's feeding time.

4. Once you've identified all of the rules, including the triggers, associated thoughts, and resulting resolutions, then the next step is to organize them into a hierarchy from least to most disturbing. Using a SUD (Subjective Units of Discomfort) scale of 0 (no discomfort) to 10 (maximum discomfort), rate each rule according to how disturbed you'd feel to not comply with your anxiety monster's demands either by delaying or overlooking each of the rules. If you cut down on the excessive time and standards of cleaning and sanitizing all bottles, how distraught would you be from 0 to 10? If you feed baby your natural breast milk instead of formula milk without purposely visualizing their joyful play during feedings, how uncomfortable would you be 0–10? To help you organize these rules, I've included my own chart below.

My Experience

We left the hospital five days later and were relieved that Tristan had gotten strong enough in the NICU by then to leave with us. The initial days and weeks were a blur with around-the-clock nursing, pumping, diaper changes, cleaning and sanitizing bottles, taking random thirty-minute power naps, then restarting the whole process again with each baby. Despite the insanity of those early days, it was still manageable. Juggling multiple tasks under very little sleep was not new to me. What wasn't manageable was the unexpected return of my OCD.

Within the first week upon returning home, OCD reared its ugly head once again. My fear was that I would love one twin more than the other, and in some weird OCD way, would cause harm to their emotional development. To neutralize this intrusive obsession, I made myself crazy by ensuring that everything I did for one of the boys was exactly the same as the other. From something as mundane as how each bottle gets scrubbed to the more complicated measurement of skin-to-skin contact, OCD dug its claws into just about every facet of motherhood. Breastfeeding became the most taxing task as I attempted to quantify the exact amount of milk each infant got during their feedings with some senseless mathematical formula. Length of time x Rate of sucking x Milk production x Time of day = You get the idea of the insanity of OCD.

To make matters even more exhausting, I spent each night checking my memory bank for the number of times I thought of Tristan compared to Dash, evaluating the content and emotional context of each thought. All of this was in vain, just to say I loved them equally. I drove myself insane. Or put more correctly, OCD drove me insane and robbed me of the blissful joy I had dreamed of throughout my pregnancy. Aside from these unexpected fears, I also had some of the more common postpartum OCD symptoms, such as excessive handwashing, sanitizing bottles, and checking for our boys' safety: The skin on my hands was once again chapped, cracked, and raw. Clean bottles couldn't touch anything unsanitized. And I had to touch my babies' chests to make sure I felt them rise and fall. Seeing that they were breathing while asleep wasn't enough. This was how I spent the first few months of motherhood—bliss turned into torment.

Once I confided in my mentor about these struggles that disturbed the precious moments with my boys, a light bulb finally illuminated over my OCD monster's hidden pranks. I knew that in order to reclaim my mind free from OCD's claws, I had to begin collecting the data of its rules that I had been mindlessly following.

Triggers	Intrusive Thoughts	Escape Behaviors	SUD (0-10)
Nursing	If one twin gets less milk, then his development will be affected.	Take careful notes, use timer, and calculate rate of sucking.	8
Skin-to-Skin	If I gaze at one twin with more loving feelings, then I will be less emotionally connected to the other.	Only have the same positive images and feelings with each twin.	7
Boys sleeping	I must leave my hands on their chests to feel them breathing while asleep.	Staying awake while babies slept.	6
Nighttime	If I attend to my boys differently, then I would be treating them unequally and unfairly.	mentally review the day instead of resting to make sure everything I did and felt for one twin was exactly the same as the other.	8
Cleaning bottles	If I don't clean each bottle exactly the same way, then one twin may get an infection.	Count the number of times each bottle part is scrubbed. Use the sanitizer's timer and place each item in it in the exact same position.	5
Hand-washing	If I don't wash my hands with hot running water and use nontoxic, antibacterial soap, then I will get the boys sick.	Wash hands and arms in hot water with organic antibacterial soap, thoroughly scrubbing underneath each fingernail before handling twins or anything they would touch.	5

Taking the time to gather the needed information can definitely feel tedious, especially when you're sleep-deprived and juggling multiple demands of mom life. For me, I kept two notepads readily opened on a table. One that recorded my boys' sleep, feeding, and diaper schedule while the other was dedicated to detecting and strategizing for my OCD's annihilation. If you're also a mom who feels it's important to document stats of every feeding, diaper change, and sleep, then recording these anxiety rules that only disrupt the blissful bond with baby is just as (if not more) imperative. Having this detailed intel is essential to attack your anxiety monster in the next steps. Think of this as your master plan to reclaim your mind, time, and bond with baby.

Living a Courageous Life Through Exposures

There are two main types of exposures: imaginal and in vivo. Imaginal exposure, as the term implies, means vividly imagining our avoided fears, whereas in vivo exposure means facing fears directly in real world conditions. The more direct the exposures are, the more effective. However, not all intrusive thoughts or feared situations can be dealt with directly. For those where direct in vivo exposures would be impractical or unethical, imaginal exposures are used instead. You may be wondering, how do you distinguish which triggers fall along that line? Ask yourself, *If I don't follow one of the rigid anxiety rules and do the opposite instead, would it result in direct injury? Or if I purposely engage in the same activity observed in the intrusive, frightening images, would it cause direct harm?*

For instance, if one of the rules is cleaning and sterilizing baby bottles with exorbitant procedures and you simply hand-washed them with warm soapy water before air-drying them in an uncomplicated manner, would that result in direct injury? Likely not. Since the risk is low here, the most efficient way to tackle this worry is through in vivo exposure. On the other hand, if one of your avoided intrusive images involves baby drowning in the tub, of course, it would be unethical and harmful to let baby drown. In such cases, imaginal exposures are used instead to tackle the dreaded images.

For some mamas or situations where the triggered anxiety is overly intense at first, going the in vivo route may be too overwhelming to start even though it wouldn't lead to direct harm or injury. In these instances, exposures can begin imaginally before attempting them in vivo as tolerance gradually develops. The secret is being aware of your own true intentions to prevent deceiving yourself from the arduous task of in vivo exposures in favor of imaginal exposures. Thus, the ideal goal is to reach in vivo exposures as quickly as possible when warranted and appropriate. Delaying this process will only maintain your anxiety monster's power and keep you from reaching your desire to connect authentically with your little love.

Are there risks involved when practicing these exposures? The purpose of any exposure exercise is not to put you or your lovebug deliberately in harm's way. Instead, the aim is to put those intrusive, frightening worries to the test while lessening the rigidity of the consequential anxious rules. Thoughts in imaginal exposures are only fueled by the meaning and associations we give them. On their own, thoughts are weightless and impotent without our steering of them. Remember the yellow duck experiment? The more you're actively engaged in visualizing that yellow duck, the less visible it becomes. Essentially, you're numbing your sensory input from the details of the images with repeated focus. This is why exposures work and have a paradoxical effect.

To annihilate your anxious monster, follow these steps to implement exposures and continue expanding your comfort through discomfort. We'll first highlight principles of in vivo exposures and then expand to imaginary exposures for those situations or fears where a less direct approach is warranted.

In Vivo Exposures

1. In vivo exposure essentially means facing your intrusive, frightening thoughts in real life. To structure this, we'll start with the feared situation or trigger with the lowest SUD rating according to the rules hierarchy developed earlier. For instance, if the avoided situation is feeding baby with your own breastmilk for fear that it may be contaminated with toxins, then the exposure would involve actually feeding baby with your breastmilk. Remember in vivo exposures are used for situations where injury is unlikely. If instead the fear is baby drowning, we wouldn't intentionally drown

baby. Imaginal exposures would be used for such situations. However, there may be idiosyncratic practices around bathing your little one to prevent drowning that may be excessive and irrational. For instance, one rule might be to keep your attention constantly on baby's head during baths without looking away for even a second to reach for soap or a towel. We would eliminate or modify those rigid rules to normalize procedures around bathing itself.

2.   The purpose of exposures is to build tolerance to the feared situation, which can only be accomplished through repeated practice. We measure exposures with the SUD scale of 0 (no discomfort) to 10 (maximum discomfort). The goal during an exposure is to reach a tolerable SUD level of 2 or 3 because it is unreasonable to feel no discomfort even after many repeated exposures. Similarly, it's unrealistic to not be frightened after watching a horror film even after several viewings. With each viewing, your initial shock will be experienced less intensely and the residual fright will last for shorter durations. Likewise, the first exposure will likely trigger intense discomfort and take roughly sixty to ninety minutes before reaching a tolerable SUD level of 2–3. Each time the same exposure is repeated, the intensity of your discomfort will be less and the duration to reach a tolerable SUD level will be reduced.

3.   How do you know when you're done with an exposure? When your SUD level reaches no higher than 2–3 at the outset of an exposure. Once you reach this point, it's a signal that you're ready for the next exposure. You can move on to the next feared situation within the same SUD level or continue up the rules hierarchy to the next trigger with a higher SUD level. Each exposure will give you the corrective feedback that you've got what it takes to handle the unthinkable. This confidence that comes from facing your dreaded intrusive thoughts one by one is what's needed to keep up the momentum. As you tackle the next exposure and the one after that, you'll be kicking your anxiety monster to the curb to truly protect your bond with baby.

4. Because new motherhood comes with very limited time, some mamas may choose to tackle several exposures at the same time, which is totally acceptable. You're in charge of your exposures and can move up or down the rules hierarchy at your pace and tolerance. Just be sure that you're staying mentally present in each exposure experience by grounding yourself in the situation with as many of your five senses as possible. Actively see, hear, feel, and even taste and smell what's happening in the moment without mentally or emotionally distracting yourself. Be patient with the process and yourself. If one exposure is too painful, choose a different one. As long as you continue to face the anxiety monster, its shadow will dissipate more and more while you take over its power and regain your authentic connection with your little love.

Kendall's Experience

Kendall had no trouble identifying and organizing her anxious rules. She had lived through them every day for the past five months; however, she did have trouble committing to exposures and initially refused to do them altogether out of fear that the triggered fight-or-flight stress response would be harmful to her delicate pregnancy. After all, suffering another miscarriage was currently her biggest fear and she was doing everything in her power to prevent it. Recognizing that her apprehension was shared by many women in the prenatal stage, we acknowledged her cautious care for her baby's wellness. Even so, it had to be gently clarified to Kendall that her body was responding to stress constantly anyway from the uncontrollable intrusive thoughts that naturally triggered her anxiety. In fact, the worries of another loss had now also infiltrated her time in yoga and meditation, which used to be her haven. Kendall was reminded that the only difference between engaging in exposures and agonizing through intrusive thoughts was that one occurred under her control while the other was controlled by her spontaneous anxious monster.

Kendall was assured that her exposures wouldn't be any more agonizing than the ones I've had to endure myself. Having considered these points, she was somewhat comforted and acquiesced to trying her first in vivo exposure. Since every rule on her list rated very high according to the 0–10 SUD scale, she chose the one that was most interfering and consumed most of her time: The rule was to check everything related to pregnancy and preventing a miscarriage online through medical and healthcare websites. From what foods to eat or avoid to what exercises were safe versus dangerous, Kendall had to research every detail through multiple online sources. When she wasn't certain whether the answers were solid enough, she added them to a list of questions that she brought to each prenatal appointment to get clarity from her OB. To simplify her first exposure, we had to break these multiple steps further. We considered three options that she felt most ready to tackle: (1) adding only her top three questions to the list for her OB without researching anything online first; (2) checking only one online site without also seeking reassurance from her OB; or the most challenging option, (3) sitting with the discomfort of not researching online or seeking OB reassurances, and being uncertain by not knowing.

Kendall chose to start with number two. The first twenty minutes were the most excruciating with her SUD rising to 7. Kendall felt unfulfilled from the one site she researched. She wanted more and was reminded that this was the anxiety monster's objective, whereas her goal was to achieve long-term calm to truly benefit her pregnancy. After another twenty minutes of back-and-forth rationalizing, her SUD peaked to 8, and she used the fifteen-minute worry time to manage the anxiety that was escalating from her ruminations. With that, she was also exposing herself to the fears of miscarrying because of her perceived negligence to research sufficiently. Even though her SUD remained steady at 8 following the worry time, it didn't rise any further. Next, Kendall repeatedly read each statement in her worry time while being present with the catastrophic images that surfaced. After rereading for another ten minutes or so, her SUD slowly began to dissipate to 7, 6, 5, 4, and finally to 3. Kendall's very first exposure took close to ninety minutes. With slightly more confidence, Kendall was instructed to repeat the same process with other questions that she felt the urge to research. Each exposure that she completed became less intense with lower SUD ratings and less time to reach a SUD of 2–3.

Imaginal Exposures

1. When preparing a script for imaginal exposures, the most important aspects are the details of the terrifying, avoided situation. You want to write a narrative that describes exactly what you see from beginning to end, zooming into the especially heartbreaking painful scenes and catastrophic consequences. Use present and active tense instead of passive verbs to keep your imagination focused. For instance, "Water *is flowing* over my helpless baby as his head *is sinking* into the tub" instead of "Water *flowed* over his head." Include your thoughts and feelings when writing about this unthinkable situation to add contextual depth to your exposures. The narrative will likely take a few paragraphs to complete. Keep the details on the specific dreaded scene without going off on unnecessary tangents that can be too distracting.

2. Once you've written your narrative detailing the feared catastrophic consequence, the next step is to record an audio of it that can be listened to on a loop. Simply use an audio app on your phone and speak clearly without rushing through the recording. If you become hesitant or teary during the recording, that's okay. Keep recording your natural motherly reactions and the painful emotions that come with it. The key is to build tolerance and acceptance of the uncertainties that come with life, which means facing those unpleasant feelings when they arise from the frightful thoughts.

3. When you have your recording, actively listen to the audio on a loop and let it guide your visualization as if the scenes are occurring in real life. Stay present with the images that surface, as agonizing as they are, without mentally blocking or distracting yourself. Just like in vivo exposures, imaginal exposures can initially take sixty to ninety minutes to tolerate before your SUD level decreases to 2 or 3. Try to get in as many exposure sessions daily as you humanly can with the limited time available. Keep repeating the same audio loop until the elevation of your discomfort doesn't pass SUD level of 2 or 3 at the outset of the exposure.

Once you're there, that's the signal that you've tackled this imaginal exposure and are ready to prepare the next one according to your rules hierarchy. Remember, it's unrealistic to not feel discomfort or achieve a SUD level of 0 because anyone would find it difficult to imagine the unthinkable. The SUD level we're looking to reach is mild discomfort without residual excessive ruminations or intense negative emotions.

4. Most times, our minds wander off conveniently when we prefer to be distracted than focused on the painful images. This is a mental avoidance tactic that isn't helpful. To counter these occasions, we have to include as many of our five senses that are relevant to the imagery work. Some suggestions include listening to the audio loop while browsing through photos or videos of your innocent, cheerful baby. Or even being close to baby while listening to the audio loop. Use headphones if that helps or play it out loud on your phone if that feels more natural. The goal is to completely immerse yourself into your dreaded imagination in order to decrease the negative impact of the images over time and with repeated exposures.

5. Sometimes, your SUD level may rise and fall during an imaginal exposure, though never completely reaching a 2 or 3 for the entirety of the audio loop. In these situations, using Hot Phrase exposures can be a helpful method to deliberately tackle those specific scenes that are hardest to overcome. To do this, first highlight the specific phrases in your script that trigger intense discomfort. Then, take one phrase at a time and repeatedly write out the same phrase while visualizing its occurrence until your SUD level decreases to a 2 or 3 before moving onto the next hot phrase. Keep repeating this process with each individual hot phrase until you've worked through them all.

Remi's Experience

Remi met with a reproductive specialist to learn more about her options. Despite gathering the pros and cons of freezing her eggs for later use versus starting her pregnancy journey early, she still felt anxiously stuck and unable to make the perfect decision for her current situation. Simply put, her husband had already waited two years and was eager to start their family. On the flip side, Remi had envisioned starting their family a bit later once her career was more established. She feared not being able to perfectly balance work and family until she was more accomplished in her field and financially stable. However, after receiving her fertility lab results, she learned that her ticking biological clock wasn't as sympathetic to these plans. Speaking with her colleagues also wasn't as helpful as she had hoped since each piled their own version of different worries onto her already clouded viewpoint. When Remi brought this dilemma to my attention one day, we reviewed that no decision has a perfect outcome and choices we make will have both positive and negative consequences. Rather than continuing to deliberate unproductively, she was asked to write two narratives of the worst possible outcome: choosing to delay pregnancy versus starting her pregnancy journey earlier than planned.

Delaying Pregnancy

James and I are anxiously waiting at the fertility clinic for our third attempt at embryo transfer. Our fertility specialist is looking more optimistic than we are—"third time's a charm," she says. I, on the other hand, am feeling more anxious and impatient than encouraged. Each transfer has been awfully painful, and the hormones really take a toll on my body. Plus, we have already spent most of our savings on the first two attempts and won't have the funds to try a fourth if this one doesn't work out. I am lying here waiting for them to complete the procedure, pull the catheter out, and the pain to pass. I feel like passing out. We're now in the restless waiting period, hoping to see double lines from the pregnancy test on day fourteen. I'm watching the clock tick slowly while my urine sample passes through the test stick. One minute... two minutes... three minutes—it's still negative. My heart

is collapsing. I'm trying on another stick and then a third. I'm only
seeing one line in each of the result windows, and I fall into teary
despair. I'm feeling regretful, especially toward James, who's waited so
patiently on me all these years, because I made the wrong choice.

Early Pregnancy

James and I are having a picnic at the park with our four-year-old
daughter. James takes her to the swings while I'm cleaning up the
blanket on the ground. He's a great dad, and they're looking so happy
together. In contrast, I might be looking pleasant on the exterior, except
I'm feeling miserable underneath. I never imagined being a stay-at-
home mom. Now, it's an uphill battle, trying to return to my career
after taking two years off. I'm taking random freelance jobs here and
there; however, I still feel stripped from my identity. I miss being
somebody other than "Mom" and working with a team of like-minded
people. I miss feeling good from achieving different tasks and projects,
but instead, I'm here stuck under piles of never-ending dishes and
laundry. I'm feeling resentful for not listening to my instincts and
waiting. I made a terrible choice and I don't ever feel fulfilled.

Having these detailed narratives in hand, Remi recorded the scripts onto
an audio app and was instructed to continuously listen to one for the next
three days at every possible opportunity until her SUD rating decreased to
2–3 at the onset of the loop. She then switched and played the other script
on a repeated loop for the next three days until that SUD rating also
reduced to 2–3. She also used these imagery exposures whenever she
caught her mind spiraling about her failure to meet societal expectations to
balance motherhood and careerhood equally. After a little over a week,
Remi began to feel less intimidated by these intrusive worries. From this
point, she became more amenable and confident to process her decisions
based on her values as opposed to her fears.

Embracing the uncertainties of life means accepting the existence of risks
involved in living even as they relate to our loved ones. Can you miscarry?
Indeed. Can baby die from choking, drowning, or other accidents? Sure.

These are devastating consequences that have happened to many families and we don't want to minimize their reality. Though, what kind of life would you or baby have if it's lived in a box filled with rigid rules driven by an anxiety prankster? Regrets can happen to us all because we cannot see into the future to get absolute certainty of the choices we make. Having confidence in the decisions we make and the steps we take comes from within. When you choose the path of exposures and live a courageous life, you're not only building confidence in yourself, you're also modeling confidence to your children and family. Authentic confidence just might be the best gift you can give them to build the resiliency and wellness needed to thrive in life.

Don't Listen, Don't Ask, Don't Tell

Having courage to confront fears and dreaded intrusive thoughts is a crucial part to regaining your mental and emotional freedom back. The other part is ignoring all of the rules demanded by your anxiety monster. Remember the vicious anxiety cycle? Whatever you do whether physically or mentally to gain a little bit of relief is temporary and only reinforces this cycle and the prankster's strength. Because of the intense terror triggered by worries and intrusive thoughts of catastrophic harm to you or baby, many mamas often find themselves engaging in senseless behaviors to mitigate their distress in the guise of preventing potential harm. Here are some examples of rules that many new moms have found themselves trapped repeating:

Checking or Praying

- excessive checking on your little one during sleep at the sacrifice of your own needed rest

- repeatedly taking the baby's temperature or other vitals to make sure they're healthy

- praying, pleading, or negotiating with God or a higher power to keep your loved one safe and healthy

- mentally monitoring yourself to check for inappropriate sexual thoughts during diaper changes or bath times

Washing, Sanitizing, Cleaning

- ritualized cleaning and sanitizing of baby bottles, nipples, pacifiers, or other feeding gadgets that consumes more time than necessary

- frequent cleaning and sanitizing of toys, baby gear, or anything your little one touches.

- unusual procedures around cleaning of furniture, changing table, or bedding for fear of cross-contamination or spreading germs

- excessive handwashing routine, especially before handling baby, to the point the hands are dry, cracked, or raw

Organizing, Arranging, Superstitions

- bestowing special significance to certain objects belonging to baby, beyond ordinary keepsakes

- excessively organizing baby gadgets in a specific order to prevent undue consequences

- placing baby toys or other objects in specific arrangements for good luck and to avoid catastrophic harm

Seeking Reassurance

- repeatedly asking family/friends the same question in a hundred different ways for reassurance that no harm has occurred

- overtelling what you did or didn't do with baby to make sure you didn't do anything terrible

- visiting online forums, blog posts, and articles to reassure yourself of best parenting practices

- mentally reviewing past daily events to reassure yourself that nothing bad has happened

Avoiding the Baby or Potential Threats

- avoiding diaper changes for fear of sexually abusing your little one

- not feeding your baby for fear that you'll accidentally poison them

- deliberately avoiding interactions, especially ones where you're alone with baby for fear of harming them

- not consuming certain foods or medications, even if necessary for your own health, to prevent contaminating baby through the placenta or your breastmilk

- hiding or throwing out knives, scissors, and other sharp objects to prevent potential harm or injury to your loved one

These are just a few of the more common rules that some mamas feel compelled to carry out in order to defuse alarming intrusive thoughts. Of course, ritualized rules can take on any number of forms, and are not limited to just the ones indicated here. Oftentimes when you feel an intense urge to fix or neutralize such fears and worries, these symptoms actually fall in the category of perinatal OCD. Nevertheless, the solutions illustrated here work just the same whether your intrusive dreaded thoughts about your sweet baby stem from general anxiety or OCD. You have to expose yourself to the fears and worries to diminish their credence while ignoring the rules and demands to disarm your anxious monster. To help you succeed in breaking these senseless rules that only disrupt your mother-infant attachment, follow these three guidelines.

1. Don't listen to them: The anxiety monster is a prankster. It doesn't genuinely keep you or baby safe. It only gains strength by terrorizing you into believing its nonsense. Thus, the way to regain control of your new journey with baby is to ignore its irrational antics. This literally means not giving into its demands and deliberately disregarding its absurd rules. Similar to any bad habit, the more

you practice resisting the urges to perform like a mindless puppet, the more painless it will be to continue breaking these rigid rules. Imagine how much more time you'd have for quality time to bond genuinely with your little lovebug without the anxiety monster's nonsense.

2. Do the opposite: If discounting the rules directly seems implausible at first, then try doing the opposite of what the rules demand. For instance, if a rule insists that you wash all bottles in scorching hot water, you'd use cold water instead. If a rule stipulates that you can only think pleasant thoughts when you're with baby, then let unpleasant thoughts seep through. If the anxiety monster has you asking for endless reassurances or incessantly telling and confessing your sins, then intentionally don't ask and don't tell. As agonizing as it may be to initially break these meaningless rules, the more you practice doing the opposite, the less painful it will be to ignore listening to the prankster altogether.

3. Do it differently: When all else fails, focus on complying with the rules in different ways. If it is too uncomfortable to wash all bottles in cold water, then start with lukewarm water. If it's too distressing to have unpleasant thoughts, then intentionally go for neutral thoughts that aren't absolutely pleasant. If you find it too challenging to completely resist asking and telling for reassurances sake, then change the quality of the questions and testimonies. As long as you're changing up the rules little by little, they will break while you chip along the corners and edges like a mama ninja.

Madelyn's Experience

Madelyn's number one rule was to avoid her baby due to her perceived incompetence and difficulty bonding. What Madelyn didn't realize was that she was in a catch-22 predicament. Avoidance wasn't going to help her connect intimately with her son, and without this attachment, she wouldn't have the practice opportunities to feel more competent. Instead of nervously avoiding, which didn't seem to be helpful for her anxiety or depression, she was encouraged to do things differently. After all, insanity is doing the same things while expecting different results. Madelyn didn't need much further prompting. She was already tired of feeling terrible and was motivated to feel human again. We started with feeding exposures. Madelyn opted to breastfeed during the daytime; however, her baby had gotten used to bottle feeding and Madelyn quickly became disheartened when her daughter declined to latch. Before she spiraled to self-deprecating mode, we asked her doula for guidance. After several attempts with her doula's help, Madelyn was breastfeeding.

This bit of success inspired Madelyn to continue to break other avoidance rules with babycare tasks that her doula had assumed. She tried bathing baby, supervising baby's tummy time, reading to baby, and taking stroller walks with baby, all occurring initially with her doula's presence and reassurance. Little by little, Madelyn gained confidence in her mothering role. Then it was time to break the next rule—undertaking the same tasks without the presence of her doula. Madelyn was extremely anxious on the first day without any reassurance from her doula. Her SUD was at an all-time high of 9 and she desperately wanted to call her doula. She called me instead. The thing about infants is that they're not great at waiting. So, Madelyn had to choose to either keep it moving or abandon her little one. Of course, she chose to stay the course. To feel supported, she called me at every break to inform me of her SUD rating, which dropped rather quickly. By the end of the day, Madelyn was relieved that she got through it without catastrophic mishaps. She continued to break other anxious rules by ignoring them, doing the opposite, or doing them differently. Her trust in her mothering capability strengthened that day, and so did her intimate bond with baby.

As you continue this journey to regain your freedom and authentic bond with your precious little love, remember to go at your own pace. Nothing is perfect and there isn't a designated speed to achieve the goals. Sometimes, you'll have more momentum and really kick that anxiety monster to the curb. Other times, you may feel less fierce, and that's absolutely okay too. Just be kind and compassionate with yourself and allow wiggle room for trial-and-error practice. Focus on one moment at a time and take each challenge as it comes without putting unnecessary expectations on yourself. You already have enough on your plate—and you literally popped a baby out after carrying it for three-quarters of an entire year. So, you're already an amazing mama just for having the courage!

Chapter 5

Changing Unhelpful Mind Traps

Someone once said, "Perception is nine-tenths of reality." In truth, it's likely much lower. This is why misunderstandings occur, eyewitness accounts aren't completely reliable, and our minds are often trapped in senseless fears, especially as a new mom. Because perspective is subjective, whatever we perceive in the moment is influenced by various factors. Some are more immediate, such as our mood, attention, emotional state, and exhaustion level, while others are more constant like expectations, past experiences, and even culture and values, just to name a few. Many new moms will tell you that the initial days, weeks, and months of pregnancy and motherhood come inconveniently with brain fog amplified by low mood, poor attention, anxious emotions, and most reliably, high exhaustion. No wonder we often find ourselves stuck in unhelpful mind traps during these early days with perceptions that don't necessarily reflect reality. Instead, our anxious mind is constantly attracted to any potential threat to our helpless baby simply because of our misperceptions of how best to protect them.

When frightening intrusive thoughts hijack our minds, we easily lose our awareness to a flurry of irrational thinking. These mind traps use faulty scripts of ourselves and distorted memories of the past to keep us frozen in time. While our emotional experiences provide our understanding of ourselves, others, and the world around us, our memories from these subjective experiences are often filled with misperceptions and faulty conclusions. The more salient the emotional events, the stronger and longer lasting impression they have on our belief system and expectations. With unchecked beliefs, our reality becomes influenced by faulty perceptions that keep us trapped in negative loops. Some of these false narratives might sound like, "The world is dangerous" or "My baby is unsafe" or even "I'm a terrible mom." As long as these deceptive scripts remain unchecked, you'll keep moving through your motherhood journey repeating the same unhelpful stories that disrupt rather than connect you with your precious child.

As you recall in chapter 2, our brain cannot discern the accuracy of our perceptions. It simply responds to whatever you perceive. When you perceive a threat—real or imagined—your body quickly becomes flooded with stress hormones, further (falsely) validating the salient nature of the emotional experience. To build a more accurate reality and continue reclaiming your wellness with baby, you have to let go of the distorted fears by learning to lean into the present moment, shift your perceptions, and be flexible in your mindset.

Mindfully Being in the Moment

When your perceptions are clouded by intrusive dreaded thoughts, your mind is stuck either in the past or the future. We worry about past actions and may mentally recirculate previous events to ensure nothing horrible occurs. We ruminate about future possibilities and might even seek reassurance from others to prevent potentially fatal outcomes. Each horrific image that comes to mind usually triggers another and has a domino effect, diverting your attention from reality. Very quickly, your mind spirals into a ruminado of irrational thinking that propels you to an urgent desire to protect your loved ones from impending harm. Yet, these "preventive measures" keep you in a negative fear loop that consumes an enormous amount of mental, physical, and emotional energy. Energy that new mothers lack and can instead be devoted to actually being mindful and present in the moment with baby.

You may wonder what being "mindful" means, especially in those initial days with a newborn when life just seems to be full of chaos. Making an intention to be mindfully present means deliberately choosing to exist in this moment. Our minds are easily tricked into traveling to faraway pasts or distant futures along with our preconceived beliefs, judgments, and expectations. However, allowing ourselves to purposefully just *be* in this moment eliminates the space for past- or future-oriented thinking. Without the constant catastrophic worries and fears intruding into your existence, you're more mentally free to simply be with baby in this tender moment. Remember, the reality of this present moment is all you truly have. Each moment that passes cannot be recycled, and we are never guaranteed the next moment. In essence, the time we have *now* with our loved ones is precious and irreplaceable. You can choose to be mentally present with baby— truly seeing them, cuddling them, breathing their scent, adoring their giggles and perhaps even their cries. Or you can choose to be physically present with baby, yet be mentally swept away by your misleading perceptions of looming disaster. The choice is yours.

Being anxious and being mindful both require energy. We only have so much of it at any given time before needing to recharge our fuel tank. Hence, you have a choice of how to spend that limited energy. You can let your anxiety monster take you on a disturbing trip through a Tim Burton version of Never-Never Land. Or you can abandon that anxious worry monster and fully connect with your precious love from moment to moment. I know it's easier said than done; seeing as I've been caught up in my own Tim Burton scenes on many occasions. Whenever I notice my mind being hijacked by worrisome thoughts, I remind myself to look deeply into my children's presence and this renews me with energy to drive my awareness back to present reality.

Accepting this reality means letting go of deceptive fears from the past and of the future that hold us prisoner to our rigid beliefs and faulty perceptions. It means to open our awareness to the present and experientially flow from moment to moment without minding the nonsense noise in our head. It means to flex our mindset to consider alternative viewpoints, rather than getting mentally fixated and trapped in unhelpful faulty perspectives. All of this facilitates the drive to lean into the present moment while mindfully and meaningfully "being" with your tender infant. To protect baby, you have to first protect and nurture your sacred mother-child bond by being mentally, physically, and emotionally present with them.

Building Awareness of Faulty Thinking

When you lean into the present, you are better able to recognize the inaccurate perceptions that distort your thinking, misrepresent reality, and impact how you choose to engage with yourself, with the world, and most importantly, with baby. However, as long as these inaccuracies in your thought patterns are perceived as real, you'll continue to be trapped in a vicious negative loop of one upsetting thought after another. To break free from this mind trap, you have to build awareness of your faulty thinking patterns. Though how? It's foremost important to recognize that the thoughts you have are unique to you; others may or may not share the same perspective. Yet, we're naturally biased to prioritize our thoughts and adopt them as factual without question. Hence, we tend to jump to conclusions and make assumptions without considering alternative viewpoints.

However, when you're able to acknowledge that your thoughts are subjectively individual and keep this actuality at the forefront of your awareness, then you'll begin to spot faulty thinking patterns. Having this awareness to check the accuracy of your thinking will facilitate the next step to discover other explanations that may be more reasonable before your mind spirals into another ruminado of irrational "what if" worries. For instance, you can either jump to the speculative judgment of "What if I'm not a good mother?," which is unhelpful, or come to a more judicious interpretation, such as, "I care to be a better mother."

Expanding your mental flexibility in this way will build your awareness to find alternate interpretations outside of the box and alleviate undue anxiety. The more aware you become of the specific thinking patterns you tend to get stuck in, the more quickly you'll be able to identify these negative, intrusive thoughts as they occur. Whether you constantly have frightening intrusive thoughts of harm occurring to your precious love, or you're relentlessly trapped in ruminating worries of not being a "good enough" mom, catching these deceptive thoughts will allow you to put a brake on them, turn your wheels around, and break the chains that keep you from bonding tenderly with baby. Although this awareness may feel foreign at first, with time and practice, grasping the other one-tenth of perspective will come more naturally as you devote energy to meaningful thoughts rather than lose energy to falsely intrusive ones.

Time to Flex Your Mental Muscles

With this awareness of how subjective experiences can lead to faulty beliefs of ourselves and others that don't necessarily represent reality, let's now practice a few useful strategies to actually change those unhelpful mind traps in order to break free from intrusive worries and fears.

Leaning into the Moment to Learn from Anxious Feelings

There is one key element to blocking the anxiety monster from running circles in your mind: making use of uncomfortable feelings. Emotions can guide us or debilitate us depending on how we interpret them. One mama can feel anxious whenever she sees her baby in distress and quickly jump to the conclusion that she's not doing enough. Meanwhile, another mama can have the same anxious feeling, yet associate it with the intimate bond that informs her to soothe baby. In either scenario, the uncomfortable feeling isn't the problem. The problem lies in our interpretation of that feeling. In truth, whatever you feel is your true feeling. Your emotions are real and valid. However, that doesn't necessarily mean your emotions are rational. In fact, if our emotions stem from our thoughts, and our thoughts are predominantly subjective and brimming with fallacies, then it follows that our emotions also consist of false impressions.

Too often, we let emotions overwhelm our ability to see through the anxiety monster's tricky disguise, especially as a new mom with the unfamiliar territory of protecting a pregnancy or caring for a newborn. Even experienced mothers have such worries and doubts when faulty intrusive thoughts take over. That's because whatever you believe, you are right. If you have the faintest idea that you're not a fit mother, you are right. If you believe baby will suffer from harm lest you spend every second checking on their safety, you're also right. This is the confirmation bias: a self-fulfilling prophecy that will keep your mind securely fastened in a negative loop if you let it. Whatever you believe or simply suspect, your brain antennae will be on alert to search for any remote evidence to support your expectations.

Processing your experiences in this limited way only reinforces anxiety, fear, and worry—all uncomfortable emotions that distract versus attach you with baby. In fact, your mind cannot discern whether the beliefs you hold are accurate or not without a concerted effort to check your thoughts for illogical conclusions. If you interpret the uncomfortable sensations you get from worries and fears as rational without question, then your anxiety monster will take you on a joyride to faraway pasts and distant futures to magnify your distressing feelings. If you, instead, take a breath to remain mindfully in the present and inquire about the accuracy of this unpleasant experience, you can begin to untangle the anxiety monster's voice from your own.

Rather than being pulled away and controlled by painfully distressing emotions, you can learn from and make use of them. Remember, whatever you feel is valid, though not always rational. By taking a moment to investigate your feelings, you're also inspecting the preceding intrusive thoughts for fallacies in order to break free from unhealthy mind traps. Thus, the next time you're caught off guard with an anxious, terrifying feeling, use it as a red flag to explore the validity of the thoughts and resulting emotions. Doing this before immediately reacting will slow down the fleeting thoughts, enhance your awareness of faulty thinking patterns, and lessen the anxiety that only threatens the secure attachment with your little one.

Whenever you feel an uncomfortable emotion, follow these steps to lean into the moment and learn from it while heightening your awareness of the unhelpful interpretations and narratives recycling in your mind:

1.   When you're feeling discomfort, whether it be anxiety, fear, guilt, shame, or any negative emotion, sit with it for as long as you can

rather than avoiding or reacting to it. Think of this as an opportunity to make this experience useful and purposeful. The longer you can be still with the feelings, the more you'll learn from it. As you let the feelings unfold, observe for changes in your experience.

2. Begin a thought record with a digital or paper notepad. Jot down the first thoughts that come to mind as you curiously inquire about the purpose of the felt emotions. These are your automatic thoughts—your go-to interpretations that are filled with unchecked beliefs and flawed judgments about yourself, others, and/or the situation at hand. Bring these senseless mind traps into awareness.

3. Next, identify and write down the situational trigger to each automatic thought. What happened that led to this feeling? What was the event that preceded this thought? What is the emotion signaling? What is so terrifying about this experience?

4. As you continue to observe and record your emotional experiences, you might begin to see a pattern in your thought process. Is this feeling usually triggered by similar situations? Do the same type of thoughts arise with this emotion? Use this awareness to begin connecting the dots of your thoughts and associated emotions.

Wilmina's Experience

When a mother, especially a new mom, is caught in the spiral of dreaded emotions related to her motherhood role, asking her to mindfully lean in and make room for it is often met with resistance. Still, to identify our mind traps that enable our anxious monster to play tricks on us, we have to acknowledge these distressing feelings to learn from the associated discomfort. Like many mamas, when Wilmina was first encouraged to sit with her unpleasant feelings, her emotional wall rapidly grew thicker. She didn't give up, though it took some time for her to acclimate to this approach. Once she did, she was enlightened by what she discovered and later applied this knowledge to correcting her automatic thoughts.

Feeling unprepared for a second child, Wilmina tried hard to avoid the puzzling emotions of guilt and shame. However, the more she tried to keep her anxiety from spiraling, the more prominent it became. Instead of trying to avoid her emotions, she was gently encouraged to sit with them no matter how uncomfortable they felt. The painful emotions by themselves aren't what's harmful. On the contrary, avoiding emotions can have long-term harmful effects. To learn from her confounding feelings, Wilmina had to mindfully lean into the moment and let her emotions unfold. When she finally did, in spite of her initial reluctance, she felt more than just guilt and shame. There was something else tugging at her core. The feeling was more akin to sadness and she disliked it even more. Like Joy from the Disney film Inside Out, Wilmina now also wanted to push Sadness out of her awareness. Again, the more she tried to suppress Sadness, the more pronounced it became. Yet, she could no longer hold back the tears that quickly welled up in her eyes as Sadness grew relentlessly louder and louder fighting for her attention.

Wilmina found it difficult to isolate any particular thought that would've instigated this uncharacteristic emotion, and naturally wanted to flee. Despite her hesitance, she was prepared to keep leaning into the moment with a curious mindset to see what else unfolded. All things considered, it was the healthier choice to learn from her emotions and capture the fleeting automatic thoughts that often slipped through her awareness. Knowing that her emotions stemmed from the struggles of her first pregnancy and overall motherhood journey, we used the photos and videos of her firstborn from her phone to immerse herself back to those initial days as a new mom. Browsing through those memories allowed her to finally surrender her emotional armor and let Sadness just sit within her.

As Wilmina leaned into the moment and let vulnerability take over, Sadness, along with guilt and shame, guided her to uncover potential mind traps that were keeping her stuck.

"I barely managed the first pregnancy. I'm not fit to handle another child."

"I should feel excitement, but I don't. I feel like a terrible mom already."

"I won't be able to give this baby the same devotion and attention that she deserves."

When Wilmina began jotting down these initial thoughts, she realized that they all related to her self-doubt and feelings of incompetence based on her recent experience with their first baby. She was ultimately terrified of disappointing everyone, especially herself, for being unable to embody the perfect supermom image to her children. Identifying these automatic thoughts validated her sadness and gave the tears that she no longer held back purpose. Realizing that fighting Sadness wasn't a productive use of her energy, Wilmina continued to let Sadness just be as she kept writing the thoughts that surfaced.

Emotions can be useful when we make room for them. On the other hand, when we avoid feeling distressing emotions, they'll become even more powerfully uncomfortable. If you embody a curious mindset, mindfully lean into the moment, and let your emotions guide you to your automatic thoughts, then they at least become purposeful. Ultimately, having awareness of your mind traps will help you to break free from unchecked beliefs and the resulting anxiety that can terrorize your motherhood journey. As you become more familiar with this process, keep leaning into each moment of distress by using emotions as red flags. Your awareness of this connection between uncomfortable emotions and unhelpful mind traps is what's needed to break the vicious cycle. The next step is to directly challenge the faulty thinking patterns inherent in your frightening intrusive thoughts that disrupt your wellness with baby.

Shifting Perceptions to Challenge Unrealistic Beliefs

Having awareness of the inaccuracies in our thinking that drive us to anxious feelings is a first step toward breaking free from unhealthy mind traps. The next step is to challenge the actual distortions in our thoughts so they reflect reality more accurately. To do this, we have to shift our attention from preconceived notions and evaluate ingrained thought patterns for validity. Essentially, we have to train our brains to switch gears and disconnect from negative automatic thoughts—our habitual ways of thinking that are unhelpful. The more we practice flexing our brain muscles to recognize these deep-rooted thoughts, the more adept we'll become at rejecting the senseless beliefs and judgments that keep us in anxious mode and mentally detached from baby.

We all have our go-to patterns in processing subjective information. These mental blueprints are established over time, starting with our early experiences with the world that inform us of who we are, how other people are, and what to expect from our environment. As we age, repeated experiences shape our beliefs while our thinking develops into fixed patterns. This allows our thoughts to travel at quicker speeds as they become more automatic. Although this thinking process has its pros of efficiency, there are also cons. For instance, imagine going to the market in an unfamiliar town. You have to get a map, follow directions, and look for landmarks as you slowly navigate through traffic signals and stop signs. Now compare that to visiting your local market. You can probably get there without much mental effort because you're familiar with the landscape. This is no different from our automatic thought patterns that hold our predisposed expectations.

Negative automatic thoughts fly by our awareness seamlessly, simply because they are our default construct in processing our experiences. Unlike traveling to an unfamiliar destination, there is little mental effort applied to automatic thoughts that speed through a fixed pathway. Essentially, any remotely similar scenario will trigger the same subjective interpretations unless we intentionally explore further to challenge them. If whenever baby cries, for instance, your mind quickly gets trapped in intrusive frightening images of something going wrong, it's a negative automatic thought. If baby's cries persist despite attempts to soothe your little angel and your mind swiftly spirals to the belief of being an unfit mother, it's also a negative automatic thought. Just like traveling to your local market that doesn't require much mental effort, the speed of these negative automatic thoughts have been reinforced over time. To train your brain to switch gears and disconnect from these unhelpful mind traps, you have to slow down your thinking enough to be able to diligently check for their accuracy.

Having to think slowly is initially tedious while you're learning to capture these speedy automatic thoughts. As you become more mindful of your go-to patterns in thinking and begin to question and challenge their accuracy, you'll appreciate this newfound awareness. There are various types of mind traps that hold us prisoner to the anxiety monster's bag of tricks. The more you're aware of them, the quicker you'll be at catching them in their tracks before your mind spirals to faraway pasts or distant futures. Of the many common thinking flaws, here are fourteen that have been useful for me and for many of the mamas under my care. As you read through them, you may recognize some of these patterns in your own thinking, especially in those intrusive helpless thoughts that make you cringe.

All-or-nothing thinking: You view things as a false alternative of either one extreme or another.

"If I don't do everything right during pregnancy, then I will hurt baby's health forever."

Overgeneralization: You take isolated cases and use them as evidence to make wide inferences.

"I'm having a really hard day. I'm not cut out for motherhood."

Jumping to conclusions: (a) **Mind reading:** You assume the intention of others without evidence of what they're thinking; and (b) **Fortune telling:** You arbitrarily forecast future occurrences.

"The pediatrician gave a concerned look. Something must be wrong with my child."

Reverse mind reading: You expect others to know what you are thinking without first providing relevant information.

"I'm overwhelmed and sleep-deprived, yet my partner can't tell and doesn't care to ask to help."

Catastrophizing: You automatically think of the worst-case scenario.

"If I make the wrong decision, I'll be ruining baby's future."

Magnification or Minimization: You make things out to be much bigger than they truly are, or unnecessarily diminish their significance.

"I failed my glucose screening test, so I must have gestational diabetes and nothing will help me feel better."

Mental filter: You filter information through a negative lens that you completely dwell on while ignoring any positive or neutral details.

"I thought motherhood would be more enjoyable. There must be something wrong with me."

Discounting the positives: You disregard or trivialize the positive elements about yourself, such as your efforts, attributes, qualities, or achievements.

"I would be a terribly selfish mom if I took time for self-care instead of making more time for my children."

Exceptional rule justification: You make judgments that only apply to specific cases and do not really believe them at other times, for other circumstances, or with other people.

"It's okay to keep washing even when my hands are cracked and raw since that's what I have to do to keep baby healthy."

Irrelevant connection: You link two hypotheses that are unrelated.

"I had dreadful intrusive thoughts about my baby and have now given him bad luck."

Emotional reasoning: You rationalize based on how you feel rather than objective reality.

"I can't hold baby because I'm too nervous and anxious, and feel I'll accidentally drop her."

Labeling: You assign negative descriptors rather than describing specific behaviors.

"I yelled at my child. I'm a monster."

Personalization and Blame: You hold yourself or other people personally responsible for things that aren't entirely within anyone's control.

"I'm so incompetent that I can't even do the research properly. If I spent more time, then I wouldn't have purchased this dangerous car seat that's being recalled."

"Should" Statements: You criticize yourself, others, inanimate objects, or uncontrollable situations with "shoulds" or "shouldn'ts."

"I'm a terrible mom and should have taken baby to see the doctor sooner."

Having an awareness of these automatic negative thoughts in your thinking patterns is critical to breaking free from their adverse impact. As you begin to identify them, follow these steps to question and challenge their accuracy and begin shifting your perspective:

1. Explore the list of thinking flaws and come up with your own examples from your thought process. Some may be more easily relatable than others. As you go through this list, use recently experienced uncomfortable emotions to uncover the associated mind trap from this list.

2. Determine the thinking flaw inherent within each previously identified trigger and automatic thought and write it down next to it. If there are multiple mind traps at play, pinpoint the two most relevant ones associated with the automatic thought.

3. Keep using uncomfortable emotions to inform you of existing mind traps. Each time you're feeling anxious, dreadful, guilty, or any negative emotions from intrusive frightening thoughts, take out the thought record and note what triggered the feelings along with the automatic thought, then find the accompanying thinking flaws. Recognizing the errors in your thinking patterns will provide space for you to consider alternate interpretations and shift your perceptions.

Wilmina's Experience

After Wilmina learned to make space for her uncomfortable emotions and use them to alert her of the mind traps that were occurring, it became less painful to collect the automatic thoughts prompted by her anxious monster. She kept leaning into each felt emotion, and embraced a curious mindset like an anxiety detective to dig further. As she continued to allow her emotions to be a guide, Wilmina was uncomfortably pulled to the difficult pregnancy and experience after their first child was born. She remembered the intense anxiety from the constant pressure she put on herself to keep life perfectly balanced and everyone happy during those initial days. Now, having just returned to her full-time career only a few short months ago, the terrible feelings she would have whenever she wasn't able to meet work demands or the mothering expectations she had of herself were still very fresh.

Wilmina already felt like she was constantly racing against time to meet both family and professional obligations, so the thought of the additional time and energy required for a new infant was terrifyingly unthinkable. In fact, with her first child finally turning one, she was just beginning to feel some reprieve from the constant demands of the postpartum days. Now having a bit more breathing room, she couldn't fathom returning to that frenetic state with a new baby; however, she knew her husband, Matt, wanted another child, and deep down, she believed that she did too. She just never imagined that she would be pregnant again in her late thirties after such difficulty and delay conceiving their first.

Honoring her authentic vulnerability, for Wilmina, it was time to determine the thinking flaws inherent in these thoughts to process her distressing emotions further. While mindfully leaning into the felt emotions, Wilmina used a thought record to visually shift her perceptions to a place of understanding and acceptance.

Situational Trigger	Automatic Thought	Emotional Reaction	Thinking Flaws
Getting pregnancy result	*I barely managed baby #1. I won't be able to handle another child.*	Disbelief, anxiety, fear	1. Jumping to conclusions 2. Overgeneralization
Sharing the news with Matt	*I should feel excitement, but I don't.*	Anxiety, guilt, sadness	1. Should statement 2. Personalization & blame
Recalling postpartum days from first baby	*I feel like a terrible mom already.*	Shame, grief	1. Emotional reasoning 2. Labeling
Imagining life with second baby	*I won't be able to give this baby the same devotion and attention that she deserves.*	Frustration, overwhelmed, guilt	1. Jumping to conclusions
Trying to balance work & family	*I'll be incompetent professionally and personally.*	Fear, anxiety, guilt	1. Jumping to conclusions 2. All-or-nothing
Trying to balance work & family	*Everyone will be upset and I'll be a disappointment to everyone.*	Shame, overwhelmed, sadness	1. Magnification 2. Jumping to conclusions

If you find this task challenging or you're having a difficult time identifying the thinking flaws, don't worry. Any new skill requires practice to develop, and learning to shift long-standing thinking habits will take time. As you become more familiar with this process and begin to gather irrational automatic thoughts, refer back to the list to identify the culprit to the intrusive thoughts that keep you mentally stuck. With this knowledge at hand, you'll be more prepared to build flexibility into these thoughts.

Entertain Alternate Possibilities to Build a Flexible Mindset

Is the glass half empty or half full? How you perceive each scenario reflects your mindset and results in the corresponding emotions. When baby cries, does your mind automatically jump to frightening intrusive images of harm or catastrophic outcomes that fill your emotions with anxiety and dread? Or do you perceive baby's cries as bonding opportunities to learn how to gauge your little one's communication efforts? Each of these interpretations will result in different feelings and bonding experiences. If forming a strong and healthy relationship with your loved one is a priority, then building a flexible mindset to entertain alternate interpretations is key.

Remember, whatever you perceive, you are right. It's all in the eye of the beholder. On the other hand, developing a flexible mindset means you have to zoom out to perceive the forest for the trees. When you're caught up in the details of startling intrusive thoughts or upsetting situations, your emotions tend to spiral to disturbing places as your vision gets blindsided. Perceiving reality from multiple angles will facilitate the bigger picture approach and offer other possibilities to interpret the scenario. In turn, having the option to consider things in new or diverse ways will pause the racing automatic thoughts, limit the overpowering emotions that follow and help you challenge the faulty mind traps through new clearer lens.

Not only does flexible thinking break rigid interpretations and distorted beliefs about ourselves, others, and the world, having this agile brain power also helps you adapt to uncertainty and regulate overwhelming feelings of distress—all relevant components of new motherhood. The next time alarming intrusive thoughts about baby invade your mind or you begin to ruminate over endless catastrophic "*what ifs*," acknowledge these worries as the anxiety monster's tricks to rob you from a healthy mother-child dynamic. To disrupt this cycle and nurture a meaningful relationship with your precious love, train your mind to challenge the automatic thoughts. Uncover these deeply embedded scripts filled with a lifetime of unchecked beliefs. Practicing to perceive the glass as half full instead of half empty empowers you to approach your worries with resilience rather than defeat. As you become more proficient at shifting your attention away from the false intrusive narratives to embrace other explanations, you'll be less restricted by the negative mental loop and be more mindfully present to bond authentically with baby.

Being aware of these mental connections allows you to interrupt negative thought cycles and reorient yourself to being present with baby. To build flexibility in your mindset, the following steps will help you to zoom out of rigid lenses and discover alternate interpretations necessary for your wellness:

1. From the thought record of situational triggers, automatic thoughts, and associated mind trap(s), try to find other interpretations that might possibly explain the trigger to your alarming thoughts and worries. For instance, if baby is crying, what are some common reasons babies cry? If baby is crying inconsolably, does it necessarily mean that something terrible or even irreversible has happened, or is it absolutely accurate to believe that you're an unfit mother?

2. Thinking from a curious mind like a detective, try to discover as many alternate explanations as possible to practice flexibility in interpreting situations from multiple perspectives. Keep the situational trigger in mind as you determine specific reasons for what just happened. As different interpretations arise, some will resonate more than others. Write down the one that fits reality most accurately that is also free from further thinking flaws.

3. Avoid quickly replacing one negative automatic thought with another positive automatic thought. Instead of simply replacing "I'm an unfit mother" with "I'm a fit mother," with which is just another label, try to ascertain a more specific rationale without bias toward one direction or the other. The more deeply

thought-out the explanation, the more confidence you'll have at accepting the new interpretation.

4. If you find it difficult to adopt a different interpretation, don't give up. Changing habits whether physical or mental takes time. Keep using your uncomfortable emotions to guide you to these mind traps, then do your best to reflect upon an understanding that better explains the trigger or what happened. Your faulty thinking patterns didn't develop overnight. Neither will a healthier mindset. Be patient with yourself.

Wilmina's Experience

Throughout her first trimester with baby number two, Wilmina used the thought record often whenever an uncomfortable emotion surfaced and especially when she felt mentally stuck. To continue the progress and build a flexible mindset, we related back to the Disney film Inside Out when Joy finally realized the harmony that Sadness brought and accepted her into the existence that is real living. Likewise, rather than denying Sadness space, Wilmina recognized that it was a powerful emotion that connected her heart to her children. Having a firmer grasp of her upsetting feelings, she continued to approach her thought record from a curious mind to gather other possible interpretations to replace the ones her worried mind created.

To make it a habit, Wilmina continued to use anxious feelings as a signal that automatic thoughts likely slipped through. When she wasn't able to identify a specific thought, yet felt mentally trapped, she learned to detect potential triggers during her day-to-day encounters that might have contributed to the felt emotion. The more she perceived each moment for what it was, the more she was able to detach herself from irrational mind traps. Rather than letting unfounded beliefs take her on dizzying joyrides, Wilmina found the value from these alternate perspectives to be more constructive and meaningful. She still had her reservations about having a second child, naturally so. However, sadness no longer dominated her emotions.

Situational Trigger	Automatic Thought	Emotional Reaction	Thinking Flaws	Alternative Perspective
Getting pregnancy result	*I barely managed baby #1. I won't be able to handle another child.*	Disbelief, anxiety, fear	1. Jumping to conclusions 2. Overgeneralization	*I now have experience managing one child that can prepare me for another child.*
Sharing the news with Matt	*I should feel excitement, but I don't.*	Anxiety, guilt, sadness	1. Should statement 2. Personalization and blame	*Many women feel emotions other than excitement, and my hesitations are just as valid.*
Recalling postpartum days from first baby	*I feel like a terrible mom already.*	Shame, grief	1. Emotional reasoning 2. Labeling	*I feel terrible because I want to be a great mom. It doesn't mean I'm terrible.*
Imagining life with second baby	*I won't be able to give this baby the same devotion and attention that she deserves.*	Frustration, overwhelm, guilt	1. Jumping to conclusions	*I cannot predict the future and can only do my best to give what I can.*

Situational Trigger	Automatic Thought	Emotional Reaction	Thinking Flaws	Alternative Perspective
Trying to balance work & family	I'll be incompetent professionally and personally.	Fear, anxiety, guilt	1. Jumping to conclusions 2. All-or-nothing	I can take more time to return to work if I need to.
Trying to balance work & family	Everyone will be upset and I'll be a disappointment to everyone.	Shame, overwhelm, sadness	1. magnification 2. Jumping to conclusions	No one has actually voiced being disappointed. This can be an opportunity to figure out a better arrangement.

The goal is to identify the faulty mind traps and revalue them to represent reality more accurately. Rather than ruminating and giving more meaning to the distorted thoughts than what they're worth, or overvaluing the resulting big emotions with grief, keep leaning into the moment with the uncomfortable feelings to work through the thinking flaws. As long as you're flexing your brain muscles to push through old mental habits, you'll be fostering a more flexible mindset with healthier thinking pathways. Practice creates habit and this habit can become a powerful mental tool that delivers the maternal wellness needed to mindfully be with your little lovebug. Now that you're armed with specific strategies to directly tackle dreaded intrusive thoughts, we're ready to move into Part III, where you'll learn to maintain your wellness for the long haul through a more tenable, stressless mom life—one that doesn't include your anxious monster's constant insults.

CONSTRUCT YOUR PLAN FOR LONG-TERM WELLNESS

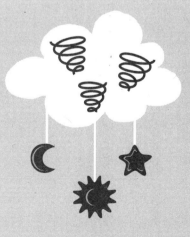

Chapter 6

Dismantling Your Perfect-Household Disease

A mother's work is never done. Literally. Our job is the most underappreciated, underpaid, misunderstood, and unacknowledged. The responsibilities of motherhood don't end when the workday ends. It is all-consuming, 24/7. There are no sick days even when you're sick and there are no vacations even when you're on vacation. Not only are we expected to be everywhere all at once and be everything to everyone but we, ourselves, actually also chant this credulous mantra and believe the ground will fall out from under us if we don't comply.

We have essentially attached ourselves to a value system that isn't only untenable—it's a path that will eventually break us, making room for intrusive, upsetting thoughts and worries. How did this happen? It's called the *invisible load*: the unrecognized mental and emotional burden we carry that underlies centuries of cultural conditioning. It has resulted in gender gaps that still largely remain today and affect how we and others value the role of mothers.

The preceding chapters provided you with insights and tools to stop the paradoxical spiral of anxiety whenever the shallow anxiety monster creeps up. Still, that was only scratching the surface. Being a new mom, to fully embrace maternal wellness and effectively stifle discouraging intrusive thoughts, you'll have to dig deeper to establish a healthier approach early on—one that is more sustainable.

Remember, your anxiety monster tackles whatever it is that you deeply care about. As a mother, especially a new mama, one thing we want most is to be the "perfect mom" to our baby and family. Despite knowing this ideal isn't realistic, unfortunately, many moms still believe that being a "good enough mom" just isn't, well, good enough. Thus, to truly lessen or even eliminate the trivial worries and anxious thoughts related to your motherhood experience, you have to delve to underlying core beliefs and fears of what it means to be an "imperfect mom." Once you've uncovered this taboo reality and the harmful consequential effects from seeking perfectionism, you too can start to implement more viable and practical job responsibilities of mom life without the constant anxiety and worries that stem from our imperfect self-image.

The Invisible Mental Load

The invisible load is the logistical, mental, physical, and emotional behind-the-scenes work that no one else sees. It is all the extra work that women take on to maintain a smooth running household and ensure everyone is nurtured and protected. It is the constant remembering that's required to keep all moving parts in a family flowing efficiently day-to-day. It is the subtle tasks, such as keeping track of important dates and events, coordinating appointments and schedules, organizing family activities and logistics, overseeing your child's daily itinerary and requirements, and managing household needs like groceries, supplies, cleaning, and repairs. It is the stress that mothers carry on our shoulders that keeps us up at night and that leads to guilt and anxiety when we aren't able to be everything and everywhere. It is what results in blurred boundaries and our loss of identity because we try to be everything to everyone and everywhere all at once.

Does this mean that fathers don't have an invisible workload or don't care enough to be involved? Yes and no. Many men today do indeed help out more than ever before; however, according to research, women still take on 60 percent more household maintenance work (Besen-Cassino and Cassino 2014). In fact, women are responsible for the vast majority of the invisible load even when both partners work full-time, and even when she is the primary income earner (Doan and Quadlin 2018). It'd be easy to justify this gender gap by blaming fathers who only care to do the bare minimum, leaving all the extra workload for mothers. However, that doesn't exactly paint an accurate picture. To describe this inequity fairly, we need to unpack the complex phenomenon behind a woman's unconscious inclination to carry the invisible load automatically.

Your Perfect-Household Disease

Like many mamas, you probably do the bulk of the gatekeeping in your household. You're the one who remembers to make doctor's appointments; research baby gear, toys, and gadgets; book flights and hotels; coordinate childcare duties; schedule the handyman; inquire on pregnancy and baby enrichment classes; RSVP to birthday invites; submit bill payments; respond to daycare emails; and anticipate everyone's needs. You're the one who remembers to buy more paper towels, milk and bread, dog treats, baby clothing and diapers, light bulbs, cleaning supplies, and birthday cards. You're also the one who knows where everything is kept—because you're the one who does the organizing and arranging. Most tiresomely, you're the one who everyone goes to for information, assistance, solutions, and reassurance even when you're not physically available and your partner might be standing right there. Alas, you hand your partner a ready-made to-do list to attend to at his convenience while you're exhausted from the invisible worry work because you suffer from the "perfect-household" disease.

Why do mothers hold ourselves to this level of perfectionism? To our detriment, we've been raised to internalize our self-worth with our flawless ability to maintain a perfect home and meet the needs of others. Through centuries of conditioning, little girls have been praised for being sweet, helpful, and well-mannered. Research indicates that parents with both daughters and sons will assign 25 percent more household chores on average to their daughters while compensating them 10-30 percent less in allowances (Bianchi et al. 2012). This remarkable difference in how we regard girls and what we expect of them illustrates the insidious gender bias that has led to our identity being tied to selfless and nurturing roles. Essentially, women have been socialized from childhood to take on more household chores, put the needs of others before our own, and regard our efforts and contributions with less value. For mothers and women universally, this has resulted in the invisible load that we have been conditioned to carry without even realizing it and it has created an expectation that we will always be available for our families regardless of our own needs or desires.

On the other hand, men, in general, haven't been conditioned to attach the same values to their identity. In fact, while daughters are more likely to be praised and rewarded for attending to household chores, parents not only assign fewer chores to their sons, they are also pardoned more often for incomplete chores (Coltrane 2000). Since chores provide our children with practice and preparation for adult life, the gender bias simply perpetuates generation after generation. Hence, even for a father who strives for a tidy, clean home, his sense of responsibility will tend to be less and his relationship with domestic labor will have a lower value system. Since a man's commitment to household responsibilities has been culturally conditioned at different levels starting in childhood, assuming he'll innately meet our standards of domestic perfection and join us in shouldering the invisible load may be oversimplifying reality. This isn't because he doesn't care about the equal share of labor, he just hasn't been raised to care to the same degree or attach the same meaning to his identity.

Socially, a father who attends to minimal household chores and childcare is still perceived as a "good" father whereas a mother would be judged as a "bad" mother (Doan and Quadlin 2018). No wonder many mamas are often trapped in unhealthy, intrusive thoughts and worries that lead to feelings of anxiety and guilt for their inability to be everything and everywhere, literally. To change this gender bias and empower mothers to embrace an imperfect household, it is imperative to share the workload, both visible and invisible. Just imagine what you'll also be role modeling to baby: a more balanced, compassionate, and equitable household.

Time to Flex Your Mental Muscles

To create a more tenable and stressless reality, use these key strategies to uncover your invisible mental load and share the household responsibilities. As you recognize the core beliefs that bind you to your perfect-household disease, you'll be more ready to correct this biased living and model a more meaningful relationship based on wellness for your innocent little one.

Sharing the Invisible Load

As a result of generations of social conditioning, you inherently burden yourself with the invisible worry work while your family automatically expects you to. From all of the logistical coordination in the background to having to remember everything related to running a household, you do it all quietly until resentment sets in for the lack of appreciation from your family. Not only do you feel undervalued, underpaid, and under-acknowledged, it's also never enough. Just like the Giving Tree, as long as you're giving, everyone will want more of you to be more of everything and be more everywhere. You involuntarily oblige because if not you, then who? Well, no wonder many mamas are exhausted, anxious, at the brink of burnout, and sometimes display our own emotional outburst. Whether you have a career outside the home or not, you certainly have multiple full-time jobs inside the home on top of the invisible load.

Nonetheless, if fathers tried to shoulder more of your invisible responsibilities, how would you honestly feel? Would you be relieved and less stressed, or would you be equally worried that your partner wasn't worrying to the same degree about the same things that you would? Would you constantly check to make sure your partner was attending to tasks in the right way according to your instructions, or would you simply hand over the responsibility and trust that they'll figure it out? If you have mixed feelings about sharing the invisible burden with your partner or others, even if they willingly volunteer, you're not alone. Many moms I've worked with often believe that it'll just be easier to do it themselves than to delegate a task to someone else who might do it wrong, or not to their satisfaction. Hence, our dilemma: not only have we internalized this sexist bias, we also tend to propagate this deceptive gender paradigm.

Unless you want to continue being your household's probation officer, checking on your partner or anyone else repeatedly only implies that you don't trust them to complete tasks to your expectations. Judging their way of handling responsibilities will likely escalate both your anxieties and diminish their attempts to shoulder the invisible load with you. Similarly, constantly stepping in to manage other family members' duties only infers that you don't have faith in them to handle it, which weakens their belief in themselves and maintains their reliance on you. Regularly fixing your family's dilemmas when they are capable of solving their own problems only robs them of these learning opportunities that build self-sufficiency, confidence, and resilience. All of which preserves your invisible burden and anxiety, while propagating the generational gender gap. At the end of the day, you are your family's role model. Are you demonstrating mental wellness and conveying the importance of sharing household responsibilities equally because that's what families do? Or are you implicitly communicating that only you can do it perfectly right because they aren't adequate or capable?

To honor your maternal wellness for the long run, you have to make the invisible load that you ultimately carry more visible. You have to truly do less by sharing more than just chores from a ready-made to-do list. You have to let your partner and family in on the invisible logistical, mental, physical, and emotional behind-the-scenes responsibilities. You have to accept your partner's way of managing household obligations imperfectly without adding your criticizing comments or giving your disapproving side-eye glances. You have to guide your family, then hold them accountable for the mental load that they expect of you. Most importantly, you have to authentically convey that you trust your family to handle their own share of the invisible load.

To free yourself from the physical, logistical, and emotional labor that add unnecessary stress and worries to your new mothering role, follow these steps to help you uncover your worry work and establish a plan for each family member to shoulder their share of this mental load:

1. To unpack the invisible load, use a digital or physical notepad to keep track of all the household things that you have to remember to do, both big and small, that ensure your household runs smoothly. Use a separate list for daily tasks, weekly tasks, monthly tasks, and even yearly tasks. Include things like cleaning and upkeep, meal planning and cooking, groceries and supplies, doctor appointments and daycare activities, finances and bill payments, playdates and birthdays, holidays and vacations, work and family schedules. As you go through your days and weeks, add any task that you are doing or must remember to do into this list.

2. As you make your Invisible Load List, consider and include the emotional and mental labor that you carry versus just the logistical and physical work. When your baby's childcare isn't available, who takes on this emotional burden? When your daycare needs more of baby's diapers, who steps in to address this? While physical labor is usually fixed and expected, and logistical labor can sometimes be mixed, emotional labor tends to occur spontaneously and unexpectedly, requiring unplanned time and emotional effort. Group your household tasks into separate categories:

   a. Physical Labor: taking out the trash, loading/unloading the dishwasher, carpooling, paying bills, bathing baby, grocery shopping, etc.

   b. Logistical Mental Labor: coordinating schedules, assigning chores, responding to daycare requests, meal planning, preparing grocery and supplies shopping lists, scheduling maintenance, etc.

   c. Emotional Labor: adjusting to the new role of motherhood, managing baby's fussiness or colic, handling new responsibilities or conflicts in parenting, providing emotional support when a family member has a terrible day, etc.

3. Once you have a clear comprehensive list of your invisible load, look for patterns and themes in the tasks that cause you the most distress and worry by adding a star next to those items. Is it having to spend excessive time coordinating each of your family member's

daily itinerary and schedules? Perhaps it's the mental load of having to be the go-to person for answers of where everything is stored? Maybe you're the only one who remembers birthdays, holiday planning, and other important events? These starred items take precedence to be addressed.

4. Evaluate which responsibilities from the Invisible Load List, especially the starred items, can be delegated to your partner, other family members or helpers, and communicate this in a family meeting. Consider outsourcing tasks like cleaning, gardening, carpooling, grocery shopping, or other household errands to a hired assistant or professional service. Maintain a weekly or twice-monthly family meeting to have open and honest dialogues about what's working or what solutions can be implemented so everyone can collaborate cohesively for your imperfect household to be more manageable.

Kendall's Experience

Kendall had never considered that her stress and anxiety were the result of her perfect-household disease, conditioned from centuries of implicit messages. Her husband, Rob, tries to shoulder some of their household responsibilities; however, like many families, Kendall remained the gatekeeper for all things that required knowing. Initially, she didn't mind being the go-to person. It felt good being the one in charge and she felt useful whenever Rob relied on her. Yet, the responsibilities quickly multiplied over the years as she continued taking over tasks here and there to be helpful. Except now, having a third high-risk pregnancy, Kendall felt overwhelmed and exhausted from all of the invisible workload that didn't previously trouble her to this degree. With the extra medical appointments, lab work, and weekly scans that consumed many additional hours, Kendall became absorbed by the worries and intrusive thoughts of failing her regular household obligations. To top it off, the amount of time she still spent researching online took up a great deal of her physical, mental, and emotional bandwidth, especially the questions that related to her pregnancy and unborn child.

Grateful to be pregnant again, Kendall wanted nothing more than to protect the long-desired baby in her belly. To do so, she knew that the constant anxiety she felt on the daily from all of the unfinished household work had to be curbed. She began to feel resentful toward the invisible tasks that had piled onto her plate over the years. Most days, she wondered how much of what she did for their family did Rob even recognize. Sometimes, she even felt like she already had a third child to care for—not that Rob was incapable of taking care of himself. He simply relied on her for all questions and concerns related to their family, which were exhausting on their own. The times when Rob had tried to help, he'd leave tasks incomplete to her standards or come back from grocery shopping with odd brands that she would never consider. Kendall believed it was just easier to choose her battles and do it herself than having to redo everything or start an argument. However, she also felt patronized and blamed whenever he would urge her to prioritize yoga and meditation to mitigate all of the stress she felt, all because she had offered to be helpful by taking on their household responsibilities.

Yes, Kendall felt anxious and bitter. In one of our sessions, she lamented about the resentments that were building. She felt as if she was living in a completely different reality than her husband. She felt the emotional weight of her pregnancy that required her to change her routines without empathetic accommodations or understanding from Rob. She felt trapped by her anxious monster that demanded she prioritize the wellness of their unborn child while proving that she could still take care of her household. It all felt like a test of strength to demonstrate that she could be the perfect mother worthy of having a baby despite the brain fog and usurped energy that came with reaching her third trimester. She realized something had to change because she could no longer keep up the worry work, especially with a baby on the way. When Kendall finally acknowledged that having a perfect household was part of the problem, we began to unpack the invisible load on her shoulders and identified the labor that could be shared or outsourced. Motivated to give her unborn baby the attention she deserved, Kendall was ready to dismantle her perfect-household disease and reclaim her wellness along the way.

Invisible Load List

	PHYSICAL	LOGISTICAL	EMOTIONAL
DAILY	****Keeping home organized, clean and tidied, especially new baby area, Kitchen, and bathrooms** (Delay and delegate to Rob and sister for general organizing and tidying. use hired helper for weekly deep cleaning of bathrooms, Kitchen, baby area, bed linens, and floor.)	****Coordinating and scheduling home maintenance needs with handyman.** (use joint family calendar for Rob to rely on when updates are needed. Copy Rob in all communications.)	****Being the go-to person for all questions related to household matters** (Provide instructions & let family problem-solve on their own)
	Cooking dinners 5x/wk (Reduce cooking to 2x/wk and delegate remaining meals to Rob, takeout, or meal delivery services)	****unexpected scheduling changes from Rob's work obligations** (use joint family calendar for Rob to make direct updates)	****Prioritizing house and pregnancy demands** (use color-coded calendar to allocate time for housework vs. prenatal tasks)

	PHYSICAL	LOGISTICAL	EMOTIONAL
WEEKLY	Watering house plants weekly (Neighbor volunteered)	**Keeping up household & baby supplies shopping list weekly (Involve Rob, and other helpers to use shopping list app)	**Feeling resentful due to invisible load (Have dialogue with Rob for solutions to reduce workload. Seek couples counseling for additional support.)
	Organizing supply deliveries weekly (Sister volunteered)	**meal planning & grocery list weekly (use prepared meal delivery services. Everyone to use shared grocery list app for organization.)	**Feeling unsupported by partner for his lack of changes to accommodate prenatal adjustments (Have dialogue with Rob for solutions to increase empathy. Seek couples counseling for additional support.)
	Grocery shopping weekly (use grocery delivery services or delegate to Rob)	Communications with OB, neonatal specialist, etc. (Copy Rob in communications when possible)	Being emotionally available for each other (Resume bi-weekly or monthly dates)
	Organizing refrigerator and food pantry weekly (Sister volunteered)	Scheduling and coordinating prenatal classes, social events, housekeeper, gardener, etc. weekly (use family calendar to involve Rob)	
		Scheduling & coordinating with Rob weekly (use family calendar for ease)	

	PHYSICAL	LOGISTICAL	EMOTIONAL
MONTHLY		Paying bills monthly (use autopay for repeated bills)	**Responding to extended family's intrusive expectations (Ignore when tolerable and set healthy boundaries to correct when intolerable)
		Scheduling and coordinating with monthly home maintenance services (use family calendar to involve Rob)	**Neglecting to respond to social calls/ msgs (Respond when have sufficient bandwidth. Consider social support gained vs. giving away unavailable time.)
ANNUALLY	Decorating and purchasing gifts for birthdays and holidays	Planning and coordinating family birthdays, holidays, events, trips (use family calendar to involve Rob)	

Following these steps will help you to identify and lighten the invisible load you carry as a mother. Additionally, sharing the mental household labor with your family members equips them with the skills needed to be self-sufficient, confident, and resilient. Similarly, believing in your partner to shoulder your invisible load is a long-term collaborative effort that builds trust and a more meaningful journey. With less anxiety, worries, guilt, resentment, outbursts, and burnout, this more equitable distribution of household tasks will benefit all members in the family.

Challenging the Core Beliefs That Preserve Your Perfect-Household Disease

If you could have an extra hour every day, what would you do with that extra time? Would you use it to nourish your physical, mental, and emotional wellness or would you tackle items on your long to-do list? What if you had five extra hours? How would you use that free time? If you're like most mamas, your eyes might glow with eagerness, not because you'll be taking that time to replenish your spirit. More likely than not, you'll be trying to do all of the unfinished household tasks still waiting for your attention. In fact, if you had all the time in the world, you just might be filling up that time attempting to do more stuff more perfectly for your child, partner, family, work, colleagues, friends, community, and just about anything that requires *you*.

Many moms have said that they can't shut off their minds until *everything* is finished. So, you try to do it all at the expense of your own needs, sleep, and sanity. However, trying to "finish" never-ending piles of laundry and dishes is like trying to stop a conveyor belt without an off switch. You're tirelessly scrubbing plates and folding clothes in an eternal loop of household tasks as you're presented with more to clean and tidy, no matter how many items you've already tackled. You're trapped in a perpetual cycle of domestic duties that offers no destination or sense of accomplishment— and that's just household tasks. We haven't even piled on demands from your workplace, baby's childcare, extended families, community, or whoever else needs *you*. When we include all of the things we try to do all by ourselves to be perfect mothers, it's a very tall order that no amount of extra time can realistically accomplish.

Furthermore, when we try to do it all, and are unsuccessful because of the unrealistic expectation to completely finish everything on our never-ending to-do list, we experience mom guilt. We internalize societal pressures to be perfect and blame ourselves for our shortcomings because we've been deluded to believe in the irrational supermom ideal. We put our own needs and desires on the back burner because we've been cultured from our upbringing to judge ourselves based on our family's well-being over our own wellness. Hence, you neglect your physical, mental, and emotional health in order to keep trying to do it all perfectly. At the same time, you inadvertently wind up making space for stress to build and pressures to drive you to exhaustion, burnout, and even rage.

Suffering from the perfect-household disease, you yearn to have to do less while your partner doesn't feel the need to do as much. Consequently, you excessively worry about every detail related to your child and family and negatively judge yourself when things don't go perfectly. In your attempts to do it all, resentment might take over that naturally disrupts the connection with your family and causes the experience of "mom rage" manifested in various ways. When you're irritable from having no reserves left and resort to yelling or snapping at your family, guilt ensues. When you abrasively toss the remote control at your partner as a passive-aggressive gesture to get off the couch, it's shame that follows.

These common moments when you feel stressed, disrespected, unappreciated, and frustrated by your family's lack of care while you're trying to do it all is what fuels a mother's rage. Yet, the emotional space shadowing the rage is the playground for our intrusive, anxious thoughts. This is where our anxiety monster taunts us with worries about what we have or haven't done for our child and family while mocking us with shame for our rage and supposed shortcomings. Without awareness of this dynamic, we let our insecurities driven by societal pressures fall into this trap that sustains our perfect-household disease.

Nevertheless, have you ever thought what would really happen if you stopped doing all of the things that your family thinks occur magically? Would the entire household feel the impact immediately if you took a brief break and let just imperfection naturally be? Would your child suffer—for real? Would your partner judge you or even notice? Would your household really fall apart? You can keep trying to do it all perfectly, and end up collapsing under the pile of never-ending laundry and dishes. Or you can accept an imperfect household by pushing the off switch on your conveyor belt and take the extra hour to refuel your sanity. Choosing to not do it all, not do it perfectly, and taking the extra time for your well-being is essential to preventing burnout so you can meet the demands of motherhood in a healthier manner.

Embracing a genuine share of equal responsibilities without diving in to accommodate your family or others means you have to break free from your perfect-household disease that holds only you accountable. Using this guide, uncover what it means to you to be an imperfect mom with an imperfect household in order to amend the insecurities that keep you on the senseless hamster wheel of never-ending tasks:

1. To dig deep to your underlying core beliefs and fears of what it means to have an imperfect household, start by making a list of all the things you do that ensures your household runs and appears perfectly. Use your Invisible Load List to help identify specific household tasks that you aim to handle in your idealized perfect way. Focus especially on the tasks that you wouldn't hand off to someone else out of the belief that it wouldn't be handled correctly or properly by another person.

2. Once you've gathered this list, start with a specific labor, such as "loading/unloading the dishwasher," and identify the sequential awful consequences if the task is done imperfectly. Ask yourself, "What's so terrible if it's not handled exactly just so?" With each subsequent response, continue to uncover the next deeper consequence until no further outcome can be generated by inquiring, "What would happen if it's not perfect?" "What does that mean to me?" "What would it mean about me if it's imperfectly done?" You're starting to dig up your core beliefs about yourself, others, and your world.

3. As you continue to uncover your underlying core fears of having an imperfect household, you'll notice the irrational patterns that maintain your automatic inclination to maintain a perfect image. Just like how you handled automatic thoughts in chapter 5, challenge each of these untenable negative mental traps to break free from your perfect-household disease. Determine the thinking flaws associated with your core beliefs and an alternative solution that is more reasonable, practical, and of course, imperfect.

Madelyn's Experience

Like many mamas reading, Madelyn was motivated by the idea of sharing her household responsibilities and was definitely eager to let it all go.

Having spent five months postpartum battling anxiety and depression as a single mom had depleted just about every inch of her being. After emotionally bonding and learning about her baby in the past three months, she was now more confident in her motherly role and adored (mostly) every waking moment with her little angel; however, Madelyn was nearing the end of her maternity leave and needed to find additional help. Her trusted doula recommended that she began transitioning baby care to a nanny before returning to work to ease the initial separation. After hiring an experienced nanny who was also reliable for housekeeping duties, Madelyn was prepared to step back.

Her new nanny began to take over all baby care duties and some household tasks instinctively after about a week. However, whenever a task wasn't attended to precisely as instructed, Madelyn anxiously intervened. In fact, Madelyn spent more time correcting her nanny for minuscule details than separating from baby to ease the transition. Not because she didn't want to be free of the demands that drained her. She simply wasn't convinced that others would provide the same level of attention to her baby or manage the various baby duties to her expectations. Madelyn had flipped a 180 since her initial postpartum days and had to remind herself that the goal wasn't for her nanny to carry out the delegated tasks according to her ideals in the exact same way. That wouldn't be possible given there's only one of her. As long as each task was being met and the outcome was sufficiently reasonable, then she had to be tolerant of other's individual ways of doing things.

Despite acknowledging this logic, Madelyn couldn't help herself and initially continued stepping in to handle tasks that were assigned to her nanny. What she didn't consider were the implicit messages she was sending by constantly assuming the labor that now belonged to someone else. Like any mentor training an apprentice, it's sensible to guide, observe, and check in at the beginning; however, continuously stepping in to correct for minor imperfections will only stifle the apprentice's progress. Madelyn was encouraged to also think of the values and expectations she would be modeling to her own child one day and how that would impact her child's experiences in his own world. Still feeling reluctant, we had to dig deeper to challenge her anxious monster. It was time for Madelyn to uncover her underlying core beliefs and fears of what it meant to have an imperfect household, and perhaps, be an imperfect mama as well.

Perfect-Household Disease Challenge	
LABOR	Clipping baby's finger/toenails
FEARED CONSEQUENCES	If I don't clip my baby's nails myself...
	It will be done incorrectly by others
	His nails will be cut too short
	His fingers will bleed from improper trimmings
	The nailbeds will be injured, grow back deficiently, and affect his entire adult life
UNDERLYING CORE BELIEF	I wouldn't have done my job as the mother to keep him healthy.
THINKING FLAWS	Jumping to Conclusions, Catastrophizing, Personalization
ALTERNATIVE SOLUTIONS	Show nanny how I trim the nails, then observe her doing it. Repeat once if necessary.

Perfect-Household Disease Challenge	
LABOR	Cleaning baby furniture (tub, changing table, high chair)
FEARED CONSEQUENCES	If I don't clean baby's items...
	Others won't take the time to be meticulous
	These items won't be sufficiently cleaned
	The items will harbor illness-causing bacteria, viruses, or mold
	Baby will get sick or develop a lifelong condition

UNDERLYING CORE BELIEF	I wouldn't have done my job as the mother to keep him safe and healthy.
THINKING FLAWS	Jumping to Conclusions, Magnification, Personalization
ALTERNATIVE SOLUTIONS	Show nanny how I like things cleaned. Observe nanny one or two times and delegate task entirely to nanny.

Perfect-Household Disease Challenge	
LABOR	Grocery and household items lists
FEARED CONSEQUENCES	If I don't facilitate weekly meal planning and ensure the shopping list is in order...
	Baby might not have a variety of healthy and nutritious options
	We won't have needed items last minute
	I'll have to take time to fix the problem last minute
	I'll be even more emotionally drained
UNDERLYING CORE BELIEF	Everything will be even more chaotic if I'm not on top of all things needed.
THINKING FLAWS	All-or-Nothing, Jumping to Conclusions, Catastrophizing
ALTERNATIVE SOLUTIONS	Train nanny on food items to include for balanced, healthy meals. Share shopping list app with nanny to keep track and add grocery & household items as needed. Trust nanny to make healthy baby food options. Provide feedback to adjust as needed.

Remember, doing it yourself might seem more efficient in the short run, though at the expense of practice opportunities for others and at the sacrifice of your sanity in the long run. If you want to take the load off your invisible labor, then you have to let family and others build confidence to share the household workload despite the potentially imperfect results. As long as you keep challenging the mental traps that underlie your perfect-household disease, you'll be honoring your maternal wellness for the long haul. Show others the rope, then take a step back and allow them to be accountable for owning their share of household responsibilities. At the end of the day, you'll appreciate the energy you'll gain from sharing your invisible load. Plus, being tolerant of an imperfect mom life will paradoxically give you the wellness needed to connect authentically with baby and your family.

Chapter 7

Creating Your Boundary Mom Doctrine to Ensure Long-Term Wellness

Before having children, many women had a distinct identity. We had a reliable support system of friends who shared our various experiences and pursuits. We encouraged each other when we were apprehensive about our jobs. We lifted each other when we felt exasperated with a spiteful colleague. We lent each other an ear and shoulder for those teary breakups. Like all things that evolve over time, our separate lives eventually took us in different directions. Then after having children, the burdens of motherhood leave us with almost no time or energy and we begin to lose these important connections that once nurtured our individuality.

For many women, our motherhood journey can be the most rewarding and challenging experience at the same time. Simply scroll through any social media feed and you'll find tons of photos and videos of picture-perfect families along with sarcastic memes depicting the mayhem of mommy life. We start our motherhood journey with all sorts of dreams of the perfect mom life while baby is baking in our belly. Yet, when life with our precious newborn finally arrives, these fantasies start to crumble one by one as relentless exhaustion takes over while we lose our identity, our boundaries, and our entire self altogether to mom life. Alas, in a society that holds mostly mothers accountable for a child's upbringing, we're left in a spotlight of guilt for wanting to feel more than just the demands of motherhood or resume an identity that is other than just "Mommy." Nonetheless, guilt is what your anxious mind will latch onto. Tugging at your heartstrings, these are the unwelcomed opportunities for further intrusive thoughts and worries from your anxious monster.

You're More Than a Supermom

Why do you aspire to be a supermom? Has that ambition given you the mom life that you've desired? For decades, we have been misled by society's superhero persona that depicts perfect mothers who can do it all. The media bombards us with images of flawless supermoms who seemingly keep an immaculate household, putting nutritious home-cooked meals on the table for her family. At the same time, supermoms are able to dedicate themselves to nurturing well-behaved children and doting partners while still effortlessly maintaining successful professional and community roles. We've been deluded to believe this as the gold standard of our motherhood journey: to be self-sacrificing, perpetually joyful, and never in need of help. However, when we aren't able to meet these unrealistic expectations, because we are actually vulnerable humans and not superheroes, then we're led to think that something must be wrong with us. With guilt heaped upon us for all our flaws, our mind then spirals recklessly with critically disapproving thoughts that pave the way for our anxious monster to thrive. Consequently, we feel the urge to maintain the supermom image on the outside even though we feel the exact opposite on the inside—because who can realistically keep up that facade?

From isolation to shame to resentment and even rage, unconstructive worries of how you're failing the supermom ideal drive too many mothers like you to lose their identities trying to live up to unsustainable expectations. Yet, with cultural pressures on you to do more just to keep up a perfect motherly image, feelings of inadequacy tend to prevail. When your value and identity is judged based on your ability to do it all, many mamas will keep trying to do it all while the avalanche of anxiety, worries, and intrusive thoughts bury you deeper and deeper into despair. And so, you allow your personal identity to get lost within the expectations of mom life as society recognizes you simply as a mama to your beloved baby above all else. In reality, do you really want to be a supermom when you are so much more than just that label? You had an identity separate from motherhood once upon a time. To be mom+*(insert your name)*, you just have to rediscover who you are now that you're also a new mom.

When Boundaries Don't Exist

Throughout history, mothers have been expected to be at the frontline of parenting and give their all without limits. Even when you have nothing left of yourself to give, many mamas keep giving for fear of negative judgments. You're the first one everyone goes to for answers and to fix problems big and small. When your pediatrician needs to speak to a parent, the mother is usually who they call first. When your childcare emails registration documents to be filled out, the mother is the parent who usually attends to them. When your housekeeper requests to reschedule, the mother is again usually the one who coordinates the changes.

A famous comedian once joked that if a school called him instead of the mother to pick up their sick child, he would ask, "Which school?" This blatant anecdote illustrates the widespread reality of a woman's predicament. So, why does everything related to childcare and even things that are unrelated fall on your shoulders? And why do you continue to stay at the frontlines without limits? Yes, societal bias expects you to do it all, and when you're not doing it all or if something goes wrong, you're the one who gets the questioning eyes. That doesn't necessarily mean that you're powerless and must acquiesce to biased expectations without boundaries.

Think about this. Fathers are acknowledged as "great dads" simply for being present or showing up, whereas the same doesn't apply to mothers. We've all seen some version of this forgivable error at the park, at daycare drop-off, and in comedies: A father fastens a diaper on his baby backward, or drops baby off at daycare without milk or baby food, and spectators shoot him an understandable chuckle. He gets a pat on the back for being present and taking ownership of his child while the absence of the mother is questioned. Why do we accept society's tolerance of a father's negligent mistake as humorous while we crucify a mother in the same scenario? While cultural expectations for the division of childcare responsibilities continue to be disproportionately unbalanced, it doesn't mean you have to accede to this historical bias. Adding undeserved judgment on mothers struggling to meet the mountainous demands of motherhood is the opposite of maternal wellness.

Without healthy boundaries in place, your to-do list will continue to be on constant overload as you become the never-ending workaholic and internal calendar for your family. *When is baby's next pediatrician appointment? We're out of clean dishes. Where is the toilet paper? Baby is crying again.* Whether you're a new or veteran mom, you're often the one having to answer or fix these common scenarios. Even when you don't have the answer or aren't able to immediately handle the issue at hand, you're most likely the one expected to figure it out, regardless of other obligations that may also be occupying your attention at any given moment. Without healthy boundaries in place, you will continue to be the go-to person. Unfortunately, once you're burned-out, you won't have the physical, mental, or emotional resources to connect meaningfully with baby, or anyone for that matter, and your recovery time will be even more time-consuming.

If this isn't the mom life you've been dreaming about, allow me to assure you that this doesn't have to be your everyday reality. No, we won't be able to fix this by protesting or crucifying fathers—that's not what this is about. This is about you taking care of yourself because, again, if not you, then who? Instead of crucifying anyone for the trivial mishaps that we've all experienced, what if, instead, we give mothers, including yourself, a sympathetic smile and some leeway and acknowledge the immense burden on her shoulders? Remember, you cannot change what other people think or do; you can only change what you do with yourself, including the unhelpful judgments that fuel your guilt and anxiety. By establishing mental and emotional boundaries, you'll be fostering a healthier dynamic with yourself and others. In fact, at the core of creating boundaries, you're really just asserting your right to be well from undue stress and worries without regarding society's disapproving eye. There's no shame in that.

In order to step into the role of a well-being mother for the long haul, you have to create a mom doctrine that ensures you're living the mom life that's meaningful to *you*. You've already learned the significance of sharing your physical, mental, and emotional labor. Now, it's just as imperative to rediscover your mom+ identity that truly embodies your whole self, free from societal expectations and judgments. Then, to minimize ensuing anxiety and guilt for realizing your mom+ identity, you'll have to restructure and enforce healthier boundaries with yourself, your loved ones, and your workplace and community. As you might imagine, true maternal wellness isn't static and is necessary to protect your entire motherhood journey lasting beyond the early days as a new mom.

Time to Flex Your Mental Muscles

To reclaim your identity as a well-being mother, these steps will guide you to rediscover who you are as a whole person. Having more meaningful values in hand, you'll be better able to implement your boundary mom doctrine to create healthier connections with baby, family, and anyone else you deem worthy of your limited time.

Rediscover Your Mom+ Identity

It's easy to lose ourselves to our children, to our family, and to the role of being a new mama. From the moment we learn of our pregnancy to the instant we deliver our precious baby to the next eighteen or so years throughout our motherhood journey, we become physically, mentally, and emotionally invested. Initially, we might be filled with excitement and joy in anticipation of our new role. We get lost imagining the gentle care we'll take to nurture baby and dreaming of the loving bond we'll build with our little lovebug. When we finally meet baby, we survive our initial postpartum days and weeks learning everything there is to know about our newborn. With little sleep and plenty of demands, we devote ourselves entirely to whatever baby requires at a moment's notice. We picture the day baby will talk and walk effortlessly with eagerness while we attempt to telepathically mind-read their needs and laboriously carry their little body until that day arrives.

Yet, before baby can even talk and walk, our role and responsibilities are already all encompassing with little room for escape, and thus, we lose our sense of self deeper and deeper to keep up with our motherhood demands. We blindly assume the invisible labor expected of us and continue to give and give until one day we look into the mirror and wonder who we've become. You might question your capacity to live up to the supermom image. You might question the resentment for having to fulfill that unrealistic facade. You might even question the shame you feel for not wanting to keep giving to baby, who just keeps taking and taking what little left there is of you.

Realizing the unbalanced nature of this lopsided relationship, frustration and disappointment might set in, making room for the anxiety monster once again. Guided by your perfect-household disease and supermom ideals, feelings of guilt might now consume you. No matter how much you try to be everything and everywhere, it's still not enough to satisfy baby. Acknowledging the loss of your identity to an idealistic fantasy of motherhood that's now colored with dismay, isolation, and perhaps even a little betrayal, you might question the purpose of your devotion and relentless drive to be everything and everywhere for your family to no end.

It's not that you're a bad mother, as your anxiety monster wants you to believe. The truth is that you've had to shift your priorities and sense of self, and in doing so, have simply lost yourself. Like a new romance that's filled with excitement and passion, it's easy to get caught up and invested in your romanticized view of this perfect relationship. However, no relationship, including the one with baby, is perfect, and when it doesn't meet your idealized expectations, you become disheartened just as easily.

Like a volcano waiting to erupt, until you rediscover your identity apart from your mothering role, the pressure to keep giving without awareness of healthy boundaries will eventually reach a breaking point. To alleviate this pressure and keep it from building, you have to regain a sense of purpose aside from your motherhood duties. Remembering who you once were before joining the motherhood clan and buying into the supermom ideal will give you reasons to prioritize what you need emotionally, mentally, and physically to be a relevant individual again. Taking inventory and having an awareness of your distinct desires and uniqueness will bring clarity to the fine boundaries required for a healthier mother-child relationship. Reclaiming your space to breathe and be yourself beyond mom life will, in fact, paradoxically free you from the underlying fears, undue guilt, and intrusive worries that only rob you of your undeniable bond with baby.

The journey of motherhood is a constant push-and-pull dance. On the one hand, you're pushed to dedicate yourself to the care and wellness of your family. On the other hand, to be a well-being mother, you have to also pull yourself back and establish your boundary mom doctrine to uncover distinct purpose and goals. Despite the intensity of this emotional experience, it doesn't have to be a tug-of-war and can, instead, be a transformative experience to discover new aspects of yourself and identity. To stay grounded and keep your feet from twisting and tumbling in your dance, you have to find ways to nurture both baby *and* yourself. Embracing your role as a mother while rediscovering your mom+ identity will help you to delicately nurture your needs along with those of baby and family. This next phase of your motherhood journey can be an incredibly rewarding one focused on self-reflection and an awareness of the ever-changing nature of mom life.

To create your boundary mom doctrine, use the following self-reflection guide and Values Clarification Worksheet to rediscover your mom+ identity, determine your sense of purpose and goals, and find reasonable ways to prioritize both your own needs and those of baby:

1. Taking time for self-reflection is crucial to rediscovering your identity. This means literally setting aside alone time to reflect on your thoughts, feelings, and journey through motherhood without the distraction of others or digital devices. Use the questions from the Values Clarification Worksheet below to guide you as you begin to reflect on what's meaningful to you as a new mom. There's no need to answer each specific question at this early stage. Instead, use this reflection time to quiet your mind, connect with your inner self, and to just be. You can spend this time soaking in the tub, taking a walk, sunbathing in your backyard, or simply sitting

in your kitchen. To maintain consistent progress, dedicate small amounts of time daily or weekly, such as fifteen to twenty minutes midday or sixty to ninety minutes during the weekends. Some mamas find it more productive to retreat for an entire weekend for deeper self-discovery. Choose the approach that works best for you. The ultimate goal is to take undisturbed, quality solo time to immerse completely in your*self.*

2. When you feel ready after taking time to consider the values, desires, goals, and purpose that are meaningful to you, organize them by completing the Values Clarification Worksheet. Be patient with yourself as this process as it takes time for anyone to determine their values and rediscover their identity. This is the work that will deepen your true self so you can authentically bond with baby according to your values. Use a notepad or journal to explore further if space runs out.

3. Be honest with yourself about time constraints and make sure your plan to fulfill each goal is realistic and achievable. Too often, mamas I've worked with become so overly ambitious to immediately execute their newly developed plan that the goals themselves become a burden. Remember, you only have 168 hours in a week, which means to fit some of these items in, others in the low priority list will have to be delayed, reassigned, or removed completely. While some goals might not be achieved within the targeted time, the more important thing is that you're holding yourself accountable for starting this process within the specified time frame to ensure your wellness.

Remi's Experience

Remi wasn't a new mom just yet. She was still deep in contemplation about her readiness to embrace mom life. Other than concerns about balancing motherhood and careerhood perfectly equally, she was also quite worried about losing her identity once she became a mother. Having witnessed firsthand several of her girlfriends losing their individuality after joining the motherhood culture, a small part of Remi wondered whether this was the life she even wanted. She had observed many of her colleagues get completely swept up by their motherly roles. She commiserated with new and experienced moms who shared feelings of being depersonalized as they shuffled day in and day out to meet the demands of motherhood. And her closest friends whom she had bonded with for decades were now rarely available. Remi was terrified by all of these versions of motherhood and didn't want to lose her identity to be a zombie for her family.

Like many moms, Remi idealized the supermom identity even before starting her pregnancy journey. In her inquiries with close friends and colleagues about the options to delay pregnancy, she was also probing for their experience balancing work and family since becoming mothers; however, what she discovered wasn't what she expected, and she began to doubt her own ability to do it all. When Remi was asked to consider why it was so important to meet the supermom standard, Remi responded that she wanted to be respected as a high-achieving woman. Hearing this, we acknowledged the value in her desire to be a high-achieving woman, though her identity didn't have to be confined to her role as a mother. Instead of being defined by societal supermom expectations, the key was to focus on the values that aligned more meaningfully with her personal goals.

With that in mind, Remi alluded to the various demands associated with being a supermom that she didn't want to become. She didn't want to be physically tired and emotionally drained all the time from prioritizing everyone else's needs and neglecting her own. She didn't want to feel lost or trapped in a role that would bring on resentment toward herself or bitterness toward her family. Most significantly, she didn't want to lose her individual identity and become irrelevant only to be valued for her mothering role. These were the apprehensive worries that kept Remi in contemplation mode for six months. She kept ruminating in the dark based on other people's experiences and expectations rather than focusing on her individual and mom+ values that would foster a meaningful mom life.

Even though the Values Clarification Worksheet is usually assigned for mothers to rediscover themselves, Remi was already lost before her *potential mom life even began. She needed to work through these questions to begin identifying what it meant to be mom+Remi. By exploring what gave her meaning as a whole person and not just as a mom, she was able to make an informed decision that commenced her motherhood journey.*

Values Clarification Worksheet

1. Explore what gives you meaning in each of these areas of life. How are these relationships important? Which of these areas add significance and intention to your wellness and identity? How has your experience as a mother shaped your priorities, your sense of self, and what you want out of life in these areas?

    a. Motherhood & Family

    b. Work & Career

    c. Friends & Community

    d. Spirituality & Personal Growth

    e. Others

2. Identify specific activities that bring you joy and fulfillment in each of these areas in life. What are you passionate and interested in pursuing that you haven't had time for? Are there hobbies or self-improvement pursuits that have been on the back burner?

    a. Motherhood & Family

    b. Work & Career

    c. Friends & Community

    d. Spirituality & Personal Growth

    e. Others

3. Let's determine the timeline for your life goals. When you see yourself in one, five, and ten years, what do you

want to have achieved in each of these areas that you haven't already? Organize each of the values and specific activities identified above into short-, mid-, or long-term goals.

a.   Motherhood & Family

   Short term (3–12 months)

   Mid term (1–5 years)

   Long term (5+ years)

b.   Work & Career

   Short term (3–12 months)

   Mid term (1–5 years)

   Long term (5+ years)

c.   Friends & Community

   Short term (3–12 months)

   Mid term (1–5 years)

   Long term (5+ years)

d.   Spirituality & Personal Growth

   Short term (3–12 months)

   Mid term (1–5 years)

   Long term (5+ years)

e.   Others

   Short term (3–12 months)

   Mid term (1–5 years)

   Long term (5+ years)

4.   Having an awareness of the life goals above that you desire to fulfill, how is this different from your current life? Are there roles or responsibilities in these areas of your current life that aren't sustainable or add value and can be lowered on the priority list?

a. Motherhood & Family

b. Work & Career

c. Friends & Community

d. Others

5. How will your life goals be adapted into your rediscovered mom+ identity, so you *and* your family are able to live an intentional life? Let's take each of the valued life goals and develop a well-defined plan with measureable results that inform you of how they're getting met daily, weekly, or monthly. Begin by prioritizing the specific activities and goals according to the following categories:

Imperative: Items that have the highest priority require immediate attention and action. Values, activities, and goals that are crucial to your sense of self and well-being need to be implemented first.

Beneficial: Items with medium priority, are not time-sensitive to maintain your well-being, and can be achieved within one to five years.

Optional: Items that have low priority are not necessary for your overall well-being, though might be enjoyable or helpful. These activities may have longer-term goals and may fluctuate in level of significance over time.

a. Imperative: High priority (3–12 months)

   i. Motherhood & Family

     • Goal 1:

     • Time commitment:

     • How will I know the goal is reached and how will I feel?

ii. Work & Career

- Goal 1:

- Time commitment:

- How will I know the goal is reached and how will I feel?

iii. Friends & Community

- Goal 1:

- Time commitment:

- How will I know the goal is reached and how will I feel?

iv. Spirituality & Personal Growth

- Goal 1:

- Time commitment:

- How will I know the goal is reached and how will I feel?

v. Others

- Goal 1:

- Time commitment:

- How will I know the goal is reached and how will I feel?

b. Beneficial: Medium priority (1–5 years)

i. Motherhood & Family

- Goal 1:

- Time commitment:

- How will I know the goal is reached and how will I feel?

ii. Work & Career

- Goal 1:

- Time commitment:
- How will I know the goal is reached and how will I feel?

 iii. Friends & Community

- Goal 1:
- Time commitment:
- How will I know the goal is reached and how will I feel?

 iv. Spirituality & Personal Growth

- Goal 1:
- Time commitment:
- How will I know the goal is reached and how will I feel?

 v. Others

- Goal 1:
- Time commitment:
- How will I know the goal is reached and how will I feel?

6. Optional: Low priority (5+ years)

 i. Motherhood & Family

- Goal 1:
- Time commitment:
- How will I know the goal is reached and how will I feel?

 ii. Work & Career

- Goal 1:
- Time commitment:

- How will I know the goal is reached and how will I feel?

iii. Friends & Community

- Goal 1:

- Time commitment:

- How will I know the goal is reached and how will I feel?

iv. Spirituality & Personal Growth

- Goal 1:

- Time commitment:

- How will I know the goal is reached and how will I feel?

v. Others

- Goal 1:

- Time commitment:

- How will I know the goal is reached and how will I feel?

Check in periodically to determine whether each of your newly defined goals and activities are being reached. Discover new values through the trials and tribulations of your experiences. As the dance through motherhood pushes and pulls you in various directions, regular adjustments to your boundary mom doctrine are expected and will continue to minimize anxious thoughts about baby or guilt-ridden worries about yourself. Each time you feel imbalanced in your footsteps, check in with yourself, your feelings, your thoughts, and your sense of self. To keep grounded, use self-reflection time and revisit your Values Clarification Worksheet as needed. Again, like all previous skills you've learned, the more practice you get, the more it becomes a healthy habit. This habit will continuously redefine your authentic bond with baby whether they're one, ten, or twenty years old so you won't as easily lose yourself on your motherhood journey.

Embodying Boundaries and Structure Like Team Sports

Healthy boundaries not only protect our well-being, they also honor the boundaries of our child and partner. Healthy boundaries provide clear parameters for our relationships with others, including the one with ourselves. Trying to navigate mom life without clear boundaries is like playing in a sports team without positions or rules, except you're the only one being assigned the team captain. Everyone's running around without clear direction or goals while you're constantly trying to figure out who will do what. You struggle to communicate expectations to your teammates while the entire team is confused and frustrated with your nonstop yelling. You're disoriented from the chaos and overwhelmed from the demands and responsibilities while everyone else either doesn't want to hear your hollers or doesn't know how best to be a supportive teammate. As a result, you find yourself overcommitted, anxious, resentful, and burned-out from constantly having to play every position for everyone.

On the other hand, having clear boundaries provides structure, expectations, and order for the entire team to approach the goals of the game. It helps you to prioritize your responsibilities without stepping in to assume another teammate's position, which can leave gaps for confusion and commotion. Since every player has clearly defined roles and direction to achieve their own objectives, they'll have the structure to be supportive teammates.

When you approach your family with the boundaries and structure inherent in team sports, it doesn't just serve your wellness—you're also protecting your family's overall health from vague rules and expectations. Having healthy boundaries in place will minimize miscommunications and conflicts both within your family and with those outside of it. Physical, mental, and emotional boundaries that are sensible will guide you to make informed decisions about which demands to tolerate, which obligations belong to you versus someone else, and which requests to decline. Less opportunity for ambiguous expectations within your team means less room for your anxiety monster to taunt you with trivial worries when minor mishaps occur. When you confidently know where you stand within your team, then you will also be less inclined to judge yourself harshly for saying, "No, thank you."

Having structured rules and expectations will also allow you to model healthy boundaries for your family as they navigate household responsibilities and social expectations in their own world. More importantly, being part of a healthy team helps every member in your family develop strong confidence and personal autonomy, resulting in more fulfilling relationships with each other as goals are achieved collaboratively rather than grudgingly. Above all, establishing emotional boundaries with yourself means accepting your whole self and acknowledging your mom+ identity without guilt or shame for refusing to fulfill society's supermom expectations. In essence, establishing clear and healthy boundaries will help your family become more functional while also allowing you to reclaim the sanity and wellness needed to bond with baby for the long haul. Since this is essential to your wellness, let's take a look at where boundaries are lacking in your mom life to better define the ones to be implemented because a happy mama equals a happier family.

To continue creating your boundary mom doctrine that ensures long-term wellness, start by accepting that time dedicated to your well-being requires time to be sacrificed from elsewhere. Hence, you won't be pleasing everyone, and in fact, will likely upset some initially. Just like any sports game where some will feel victorious while others will be disappointed, your goal is to honor your needs to be well first in order to have the energy to captain your team to success. Follow these steps to clearly execute the boundaries that define the rules, expectations, and structure needed for your maternal wellness and your family harmony. If a specific area isn't applicable to you, go ahead and move onto the next section that can benefit from firmer boundaries:

1. To determine where boundaries are lacking and define the rules for your boundary mom doctrine, start by recapping your Invisible Load List and Values Clarification Worksheet that you've already uncovered. Reflect on the household demands that need adjusting in order for you to achieve a more meaningful mom+ identity. With this awareness in mind, also investigate other areas, such as work or community obligations that might be depleting your

energy because boundaries are lacking. Use a notepad or journal to begin outlining where boundaries need to be established to protect your wellness, and include the following considerations.

Work: If you're a mom who also works outside the home, building awareness of the sources in your workplace or professional role that also usurp your energy is vital to determining the boundaries needed. Ask yourself the following four questions. Your responses will help you define the rules and structure to be incorporated into your boundary mom doctrine.

- What are my expected work hours and how many hours do I actually spend working? If the amount of time spent working is in excess to the hours available for work, what is the cut-off time daily or weekly that needs to be firmly established?

- Does my work bleed into my personal time with family or take away time needed to replenish my energy? If so, what are some options to minimize these occurrences?

- Does my work provide the flexibility needed at times for unexpected childcare requirements or medical attention? If not, what are the consequences if work has to be missed? Who at work can I discuss these options with to determine a reasonable plan and curtail unnecessary anxiety and guilt?

- Am I expected to respond to emails, texts, or phone calls after work hours when my attention is needed elsewhere? If so, what is the cut-off time to eliminate burnout from having to multitask?

Community: If you give time to your community, such as volunteering at your child's daycare, religious institution, professional committees, neighborhood association, public charities, or even social events, ask yourself these four questions to determine whether the time commitments continue to align with your values and fit with your evolving motherhood requirements.

- Do the responsibilities and expectations in your community roles still hold value and meaning to your identity? If so, rate each role numerically from least to most meaningful and begin resigning from the ones with least value to regain more time.

- Do you feel pressured to say yes to every request whether it causes additional stress or burden? If you are overcommitted, choose which requests you'll say no to in order to prioritize time needed for your wellness.

- Do you feel obliged to attend every social event hosted by a friend, family, or community member and feel guilty when scheduling conflicts occur? Determine the value of the event compared to the obligations already in your schedule and practice declining invitations without the unnecessary guilt because scheduling conflicts are out of your control.

- Do you feel your downtime to recharge gets disrupted by phone calls, texts, or untimely visits from friends and extended family? Determine set times for responding to non-urgent communications, delay calls/texts to those times, and defer visits to times when you're not overextending yourself.

2. Use the insights you've gained to begin defining the rules you want to establish. This means actually spelling out your expectations of yourself, family, work, and community obligations like a playbook. What will you anticipate and allow? What will you not tolerate? Communicate these expectations clearly with all involved. Your boundary mom doctrine is your comprehensive plan to reclaim your mom+ identity, share the household load with your family, limit work encroachments, and restrict community overcommitments. Just like team meetings, hold regular family meetings to review the plans in your playbook and determine which plays are working well and which can be tweaked to work better. During these meetings, ensure each family member has a voice

and have one-on-one conversations when needed to clarify any misunderstandings. Similarly, communicate your concerns and boundary expectations gently and firmly with your coworkers, colleagues, friends, family, and community members as needed. When work and family demands conflict, explore options with your supervisor or boss to find an amicable solution.

3. Consider your emotional boundaries with yourself and others. Minimize passive communications or passive-aggressive expressions stemming from guilt, resentment, anger, or other unhelpful emotions that don't firmly reinforce your boundaries. Take ownership of your emotions without blaming others and remember that other people's reactions are not your responsibility. Be aware of the implicit messages you communicate and shift negative self-talk to yourself into resilient directives to others, such as:

   • "You can figure out solutions on your own."

   • "Please do not interrupt me unless it's a safety/emergency issue."

   • "I trust you to make a reasonable decision. You don't need my reassurance."

   • "My phone will be on silent and I won't be reachable until..."

   • "There's no need to consult me."

4. Setting the boundaries with your team is just part of the equation. You have to also enforce the expectations by modeling the importance of following your own rules without unprompted negotiations. Adhering to your own boundaries communicates that they are to be taken seriously so others will also respect you and your established limits. Therefore, practice saying no to requests that are at the expense of your personal time and wellness. Keep in mind that you already have plenty of obligations on your shoulders. Thus, each additional request that you accept will sacrifice time from something already on your plate.

Wilmina's Experience

As Wilmina continued to exercise a flexible mindset, she accepted that approaching her current pregnancy from the same standard of perfectionism with her first child was the culprit of the self-doubt and guilt she was feeling. Realizing that all of the energy devoted to being her family's supermom was part of her perfect-household disease, she became more attuned to what her sanity needed to live the mom life she actually desired. Having unpacked her invisible load, clarified her values, and rediscovered her identity, she was now slowly dismantling her perfect-household disease to create her boundary mom doctrine using the same steps as the ones within these pages. Every time we met, she became more and more aware that striving for perfection to be everything and everywhere wasn't realistic or in her best interest. She was learning to first put her oxygen mask on before trying to help others.

To ensure her doctrine was implemented, Wilmina set up weekly family meetings with Matt to talk about ways to improve their harmony together. She shared her Invisible Load List and personal goals from her boundary mom doctrine; Matt was aligned with her intentions. He had also been wanting to clarify the expectations Wilmina had of him that sometimes came across passive-aggressively or were confusing to him. Despite communicating difficult interpersonal matters, both Wilmina and Matt tried hard to put their differences and blame aside in service of their joint family goals. Having better defined mental and emotional boundaries helped both of them have a better grasp of the rules and expectations of their family life together.

Wilmina's boundary doctrine extended to work as well. After meeting with her supervisor to discuss establishing more structure for workflow productivity, she instituted uninterrupted administrative days during the work week. She minimized distractions and inefficient multitasking by dedicating specific days for client/work meetings, as well as set times for responding to non-urgent emails, calls, and texts. She kept work from carrying over to family time as much as reasonable by implementing a cut-off period for shutting down her laptop and work phone. And to keep work demands sustainable according to her doctrine, Wilmina finally *began to decline additional projects that she previously felt too guilty to turn down.*

In her social and community obligations, she selected the events and missions that aligned with her values while contributing to her rediscovered mom+Wilmina identity. She responded to messages only when she had the bandwidth without feeling the urgency to reply immediately. When social requests conflicted with her boundary mom doctrine, she practiced making rainchecks or saying no altogether, and became more comfortable doing so. Most imperatively, Wilmina was beginning to own the physical, mental, and emotional boundaries and structure without hesitation, apologies, or second-guessing herself. She was finally activating her oxygen mask first.

Practicing these guidelines to establish healthy, firm boundaries with yourself, your family, work, and community provides the structure that defines what's acceptable and unacceptable to you and your well-being. While setting boundaries means imposing limits with others that may initially elicit commotion, your time, sanity, and wellness are worth protecting. It doesn't mean you're being unkind or uncaring. It just means that you're honoring your maternal wellness first. When you continue to train those around you about how you are to be treated, they will adjust and adapt to your boundaries with time as long as you're persistent and consistent. To be your best self, you have to put your oxygen mask on first before you run out of oxygen to help anyone else. To be heard fully, you'll have to be clear, firm, and unapologetic in your boundaries that teach others to respect you and your whole self. Your loved ones would much prefer you to be your best self rather than a resentful mama when your needs aren't met. Not only will creating your boundary mom doctrine restore your sanity, it will protect your mothering love and attachment with baby and family. As you reclaim your wellness on your motherhood journey, periodically revisit the rules in your boundary mom doctrine to determine changes that have evolved. Without unwarranted guilt, worries, or alarming intrusive thoughts, there won't be room in your imperfect household for the anxiety monster to wander.

Chapter 8

Keeping It Real and Stressless

Remember *The Giving Tree*? The story of a tree who gave and gave and gave whatever she had just to make a boy happy? First, it was her apples, next was her branches, and finally, out of love, she even gave her entire trunk to the boy. Except, it was never enough and the boy still wasn't happy, or grateful for that matter. Yet, the once vibrant tree kept giving until she became an old stump and there was nothing left to give. Alas, this story, although fictional, represents the real experiences of many mamas across the globe. Without foresight, we give and give and give until suddenly, we find ourselves with nothing left to give, and still, it's not enough to keep our children and family content. Now, instead of the Giving Tree, imagine yourself as the Wellness Tree—one that is well-prepared to weather the storms that naturally come with real life without inadvertently losing your apples, branches, or entire trunk.

To ride out unexpected storms, your Wellness Tree must stay grounded to your roots and core values. Your Wellness Tree must preserve your identity and protect your boundaries by keeping your bountiful apples, branches, and trunk healthy. Most importantly, your Wellness Tree must be flexible enough to adapt to the inevitable ups and downs of motherhood by keeping your foresight realistic. Otherwise, whenever you're at a low point from unforeseen demands that sap your resources, your anxiety monster will simply try to creep back into your thoughts. Thus, to further minimize these unnecessary stresses so your Wellness Tree can flourish with its parts intact, you have to prepare for the seasons ahead and brace for the inclement weather along your motherhood journey.

Planning Ahead to Honor Your Wellness Tree

If anyone ever told you that motherhood was easy, I'd be suspicious. If we're keeping it real, then we have to acknowledge that mom life is often chaotic and definitely unpredictable, especially in the early days. One moment might be calm and managed while the very next moment might take you on an unwelcomed adventure of unexpected demands. That's the reality of motherhood. You're always vigilant and on guard for whatever comes your way. For instance, baby might wake up with a fever one morning, and like a wizard, you'll have to make a last minute pediatrician appointment and cancel your day's scheduled tasks. Or on a planned evening, you might be dressed up excitedly for your monthly date night only to disappointedly change into your pajamas when the babysitter calls with a ludicrous excuse. This is mom life keeping you on your toes.

Truth is, when children are involved, you have to be flexible and prepared to switch gears at a moment's notice. Even the best thought-out plans rarely go as planned when you're a mom, new or veteran. However, having absolutely no plan at all will leave you defenseless, resulting in spontaneous outcomes that may be detrimental to your overall well-being. Planning ahead, even if plans don't always go accordingly, at least establishes a blueprint from which to improvise when last minute detours are necessary. When we plan ahead, we account for the logistical, mental, emotional, and physical stresses required of us at a moment's notice. When these procedural boundaries are clearly defined, they give us the foresight needed to keep our Wellness Tree from scrambling and needlessly giving away all of our apples, branches, and trunk at the eleventh hour.

In fact, let's consider this: If our biggest jobs as mothers are to protect and prepare baby for real life when no one else will care as much as we do, how will you achieve this if you have nothing left of yourself to give? Like the Giving Tree without foresight, you'll be more inclined to give and give and give to problem-solve for last-minute mishaps that will only put you at risk for burnout, resentment, and depletion of resources. Hence, choose to keep your mom life real and stressless instead. By establishing day-to-day boundaries and procedures that will guide you through inevitable storms, you'll be less likely to deplete all of your physical, mental, and emotional resources. With a plan in sight, you'll be better equipped to make informed decisions and instinctive changes when the unexpected occurs without reckless reactions that might leave you barren. Being fully intact, you'll also be more adept to regain your bearing even when you're thrown off course simply because you're more prepared to navigate the unforeseen storms of mom life. If you want a better way to handle the unexpected day-to-day curve balls as a new mom, then it's time to honor your Wellness Tree.

Time to Flex Your Mental Muscles

When we prioritize our wellness, we're also choosing to enrich our loving bond with baby and our family. We're choosing to save our apples, branches, and trunk for the long run when we'll need our resources most. To plan for the realities on your motherhood journey and prevent undue stress, anxiety, or literal breakdown, put these essential strategies to work. When an unexpected storm passes through, you'll be more grounded and prepared having this blueprint to guide you to practical options and solutions.

Creating Your Annual Timeline for Work-Life Awareness

We can't do it all, and why would we want to? If you genuinely want to embrace the Wellness Tree, then it's time to accept the reality that we cannot be everything to everyone and be everywhere all at once, no matter who expects this absurd existence. To secure our boundaries and protect our apples, branches, and trunk from misuse, we have to know what lies ahead that will require our resources. This is called work-life awareness. When you have awareness of the burdens that will consume your time and stress your bandwidth, then you'll be better equipped to navigate the hurdles sensibly. On the other hand, when you're oblivious to upcoming demands that may disrupt your schedule and tax your energy, then you'll be easily blindsided and pushed off balance. The most reliable tactic to weather any storm, forecasted or abrupt, is to be prepared with knowledge and resources.

Do you know what's on your agenda this week? How about next month? Taking a proactive approach to planning your time will inform you of the reserves you'll need at any given time. By creating an annual timeline, many mamas I've helped have been able to mitigate unforeseen demands simply because they already knew what else to expect. Having an annual timeline in hand allows you to see and plan for upcoming obstacles, so when the unexpected does occur, you can pivot with more fluidity. On a week-to-week, month-to-month basis, what are the responsibilities on your plate? What duties take up your bandwidth? Who and what will require your time? Are there specific months that you anticipate will be more chaotic than others? When do you usually travel for work or with family? Are there more work deadlines or family commitments during certain times of the year?

Keeping an annual timeline gives you the foresight to predict the weather ahead in order to align your expectations and adjust your schedule accordingly. When you're not flustered in the dark, your anxiety monster also has less opportunity to surprise you with intrusive worries and dreaded thoughts. Conversely, falsely believing that you have time to be everything and everywhere, which doesn't represent real mom life, will have you panicked and constantly scrambling last minute. These moments of madness are what energize catastrophic thoughts of all the things that are wrong and self-judgments of all the flaws in your mothering ways, including your inability to maintain work-life *balance*.

Truth is, work and life are rarely balanced, and striving for that impractical ideal will lead you down a slippery slope of disappointments, frustration, and self-blame. A more reasonable attitude is to accept that life happens. Being thrown random curve balls isn't overly unbearable when you're prepared with information and a thought-out plan. When you have work-life awareness, it's a matter of executing what needs to be rescheduled, reallocated, or even removed in order to accommodate the unexpected turbulence. However, when unforeseen interruptions collide day in and day out because you have no intel, these moments become demoralizing and coalesce to feelings of confusion, rage, and eventual burnout.

To minimize heedless outcomes and pestering intrusive worries when unpredicted storms touch down, approach motherhood with work-life awareness that supports your Wellness Tree. Follow these steps to draft your annual timeline that will help you navigate the unexpected calls of mom life duties while keeping your previously established roots and values grounded to continue bonding with baby:

1. Think of your timeline as an employee handbook with details of daily, weekly, and monthly duties to be fulfilled for your job role. If you had to prepare a stranger to take over your life, what instructions would you include? What appointments, obligations, tasks, and routines are you responsible for carrying out? Start creating your annual timeline with an overview of the year and begin identifying the busiest weeks or months when significant work deadlines or family commitments are all-consuming, such as summer break or winter holidays.

2. Using a table chart, separate your annual timeline by months and include specific dates to each activity or task. Use different colors for work versus family commitments to truly delineate the imbalance between work and life demands month to month. This enhanced awareness will give you a reality check of your annual obligations and that work/life balance is rarely, if ever, a 50/50 balance.

3. Add in all one-time events that need to be considered when organizing your schedule, such as trips, weddings, medical leaves, maternity leave, baby photoshoots, graduations, sporting events, music concerts, charity galas, award ceremonies, product launches, conferences, cultural festivals, art exhibitions, or whatever else

you have plans for. If an event is tentatively planned, still include it with "tentative" notated so it's accounted for.

4. Now, zoom in closer and include all recurring appointments, meetings, and tasks that are repeated every week or month, such as team meetings, workouts, prenatal appointments, pediatrician appointments, salon appointments, baby classes, car or home maintenance, grocery shopping, restocking household supplies, bills and financial budgeting, and social gatherings.

Wilmina's Experience

Creating the annual timeline is one of the ways many mamas are able to realign their expectations of themselves and adjust their schedules to be more tenable. We'd start with a broad overview of their year, then zoom into individual months, and finally focus on each of the fifty-two weeks. The end result was a comprehensive outline of their life. As we compiled all the data needed to complete the timeline, each mama was equipped with a visual of how packed their lives actually were. Prior to this exercise, few of my patients realized just how much of their time was consumed by both big events and smaller daily obligations throughout the year. Even fewer considered how much their annual timeline had changed with a child as their family demands evolved year-to-year.

Take Wilmina, for instance. She relentlessly aimed for the perfect work-life balance. Why wouldn't she, when this idea was constantly floated around social media, news articles, and her circle of friends? Not that work-life balance wasn't ideal; she just had to accept that it wasn't realistic to expect a perfect balance all the time, especially life with a baby. However, this promoted paradigm was so central to her existence that she would be hypercritical of her inability to achieve a precise 50/50 split 24/7. When we mapped out Wilmina's timeline, identifying her busy seasons of the year from a bird's eye view before concentrating on her weekly obligations, she finally saw how irrational it was to aim for the perfect work-life balance. There were times of the year when her work demanded more of her time and attention, and other times when her home life took priority, like the holidays. This was just the nature of real life, and especially, her mom life.

In fact, even the effort it took her to thoroughly complete the timeline below was an exhaustive exercise, having to outline her entire year, color-coded with specific dates and activities separated into months. Despite the tedious process, she did gain a realistic perspective of the month-to-month, week-to-week imbalances between work and life from the color-labeled timeline in front of her. Once she accepted that a perfect 50-50 split wasn't rational, or even necessary, Wilmina was able to let go of the self-criticisms and frustration that maintained her anxious thoughts. That alone was a win! Less blame and shame equaled more mental resources and fewer triggers for the rage that threatened her wellness and attachment with the baby girl on the way. Asserting boundaries around work-life awareness means rolling with the reality that sometimes you'll lean more into work than life, and vice versa. Taking the time to create this visual timeline helped Wilmina accept this exact awareness. She shared this visual layout with Matt at one of their weekly family meetings, so they both could be aware of their family demands and be a support to each other. When she and Matt worked together as a team, Wilmina felt less alone and more confident welcoming baby number two to their boundary-aware family.

DATES	ACTIVITY	CATEGORY
JANUARY		
1/1 – 1/5	Article submissions review	Work
1st week of Jan	Winter break vacation	Family
1/17	MLK – holiday – no childcare	Family
Last week of Jan	Conference proposals due	Work
FEBRUARY		
2/1 – 2/5	Article submissions review	Work
1st week of Feb	In-staff annual trainings	Work

2/9	mom's hip surgery	Family
2/14	Valentine's Day	Family
2/21	Presidents' Day – holiday – no childcare	Family
MARCH		
3/1 – 3/5	Article submissions review	Work
3/2	matt's birthday	Family
3/15 – 3/20	Conference – Seattle	Work
3/28 – 3/31	Board retreat	Work
APRIL		
4/1 – 4/5	Article submissions review	Work
4/9 – 4/17	In-laws visiting	Family
4/25 – 4/29	workshop – DC	Work
MAY		
5/1 – 5/5	Article submissions review	Work
5/2 – 5/3	employee training – San Diego	Work
5/8	mother's Day	Family
5/16	Alumni networking event	Work
5/26 – 6/2	memorial break – Caribbean Vacation	Family
JUNE		
6/1 – 6/5	Article submissions review	Work
6/8	mom's birthday	Family
6/19	Juneteenth holiday	Family

JULY		
7/1 – 7/5	Article submissions review	Work
7/4	Independence Day – holiday – no childcare	Family
AUGUST		
8/1 – 8/5	Article submissions review	Work
8/16	Kaila's birthday	Family
SEPTEMBER		
9/1 –9/5	Article submissions review	Work
1st monday	Labor Day – holiday – no childcare	Family
OCTOBER		
10/1 – 10/5	Article submissions review	Work
1st weekend	Halloween decorating	Family
10/31	Halloween	Family
NOVEMBER		
11/1 – 11/5	Article submissions review	Work
11/11	Veterans Day – holiday – no childcare	Family
4th Thursday	Thanksgiving	Family
DECEMBER		
12/1 – 12/5	Article submissions review	Work
1st weekend	Christmas/Holiday decorating	Family
Last 2 weeks	Holiday break	Family

Like Wilmina, as you continue to fill in your timeline, you'll literally see your life being fully occupied with weekly and monthly obligations throughout the year. Take a moment to reflect on just how much you do as a mama and realize the demands needing your resources in front of you, week to week, month to month. Give yourself credit for the things you accomplish and use it to reveal your anxiety monster's attempts to trick you with irrational judgments and thoughts whenever you feel defeated. Now that you have this blueprint in front of you, you can better plan your day-to-day schedule to ensure your work and family commitments are accounted for in the time that is available in any given day. Although initially tedious, once you get your first annual timeline out of the way, all you have to do is update it annually. Make it your year-end review. This will give you the awareness needed to weather the unexpected storms that often come with motherhood without becoming unhinged.

Scheduling to Unpack Your Daily Commitments

There are only twenty-four hours in a day and 168 hours in a week. How do you spend them? If you're like most mamas, you're probably over-packing your schedule with your never-ending to-do list without accounting for the actual time you're truly granted. You might wake up one morning on a mission to checking off the tall order of items on your agenda only to be dismayed as the day quickly concludes without having even accomplished half of the items on your list. Or you might wake up in a daze after a sleepless night with baby only to be reminded of the mountain of duties on your plate piled on from yesterday's unfinished business. You're feeling defeated and incompetent because you haven't really considered the actual time you have minus the hours needed for mundane tasks just to get through a typical day. Then when life flings a surprising wrench at you that throws off your entire day, you're even further behind and overwhelmed ruminating over all of the tasks that remain on your shoulders.

To manage our various motherly roles with less stress, we have to be more realistic about our time commitments and what is truly unrestricted. Imagine any given day, how much time do you spend getting yourself ready in the morning? How much time does baby need from you in the morning?

How much time do you spend on the road getting to work, running errands, or taking baby to and from various activities? How much time do you spend grocery shopping and preparing meals? How much time do you spend cleaning after dinner, organizing your household, or other nightly rituals before you finally fall into a deep slumber? Have you ever calculated how much time is required just for daily mundane tasks? Taking a realistic inventory of your daily time commitments is a real eye-opener of the little time we actually have for just the ordinary, never mind a curveball when one gets thrown your way.

Let's say you spend ninety minutes to rush yourself and baby out the door every morning, then spend another forty-five to sixty minutes driving baby to daycare and yourself to work in rush hour traffic. In the afternoon, you spend another forty-five to sixty minutes picking baby up before heading home. Depending on whether you're ordering takeout or preparing dinner, dinner time can take anywhere between thirty and ninety minutes. If you're like my family, dinner is our quality time together and usually takes a decent hour before needing another sixty minutes to clean up and remove all of the food droppings around baby's high chair. Finally, you might spend another ninety minutes on your nighttime ritual getting baby and yourself to bed. Given this conservative schedule, you've already spent about eight hours on this basic everyday routine. If you're prioritizing your Wellness Tree, then you'll have to add another eight hours of quality sleep to restore your energy and sustain your resources. This leaves you with only eight hours remaining in any given day, and we haven't even considered the time required for work, errands, household chores, emails, bills, phone calls, other childcare obligations, social commitments, date nights, me time, and the regular curve balls that we don't anticipate in our schedule.

If you're like other moms wondering where the time goes by the end of the night, well here you go. Let me repeat, there are only twenty-four hours in a day and 168 hours in a week. Are you aware of how you're actually spending this limited time? Do you still feel the need to judge your lack of accomplishments given this reality check? In actuality, you're probably already packing more into your schedule than any mortal mama can. If you find yourself in a state of burnout, it's because you've stretched yourself so thin that you're no longer effective. Just like a rubber band that eventually loses its elasticity and snaps, you have to quit stretching before you break apart from being overstrained and awash in feelings of resentment and rage. It's time for a wake-up call from the illusory narrative that you're not doing enough. By acknowledging that there's only one of you and not many hours in a day, you're honoring your Wellness Tree while kicking your anxiety monster to the curb.

Unpacking your daily time commitments will give you the awareness to set more realistic goals and eliminate the tendency to beat yourself up for unfinished tasks. Now that you have your annual timeline and are cognizant of your obligations, follow these steps to plan your days accordingly with the actual time available to you:

1. Scheduling your tasks, obligations, and events commits you to actually doing them. Dedicating specific time periods in the day to each commitment allocates when things will get done and frees up your mental space from having to ruminate over unfinished business. This also helps you to plan your days realistically since you can see where the time goes. To start, use a physical daily planner or your phone's digital daily calendar with times divided down to the minute and plug in all of your commitments from your annual timeline. Use a different color for each category (i.e., family or work) or person (i.e., baby, partner, other children, and you). If an event is set to consume more than a day, use the "All Day" option to block out entire days, weeks, or months. This will quickly give you visuals of what is and isn't available when a task needs to be delayed or rescheduled.

2. If you're a mama who tends to overpack your schedule or unintentionally miss entire meals when you have no time to sit and eat, then consider scheduling specific breaks for breakfast, lunch, and dinner. Be as specific as needed to keep your schedule realistic and tenable. Schedule time needed to attend to baby throughout the day. Schedule morning and bedtime routines. Schedule baby care and your own wellness care. Even schedule regular fifteen- to twenty-minute breaks for a walk around your neighborhood or to

have a brief moment to clear your mind. This will give you breathing room when one appointment runs into another and will provide the space to pivot last minute when the unplanned curve ball comes flying at you.

3. Scheduling a task is much more effective and productive than adding the task to a never-ending to-do list. This is because having a to-do list without dedicated times assigned to each item won't help you see how or when they'll actually get done. As a new mom with all of your on-demand responsibilities, you simply don't have the mental resources to keep referencing back to an unplanned to-do list. Plus, an unattended to-do list will only pile up with unfinished business, which is the last thing an overwhelmed mama needs to see. Hence, if you already have a to-do list, take each task and schedule it directly into your calendar. Moving forward, either schedule your job responsibilities or delegate them to someone else instead of relying on an unstructured to-do list to help keep those self-defeating, judgmental thoughts at bay.

4. Reschedule incomplete tasks as soon as you can to keep your memory storage from overloading with unfinished business. With mommy brain in full effect, you simply have less bandwidth to be present and attend to the demands of work or family. Your mind might be spiraling with the things that you still have to do instead of navigating the unexpected storms that require your attention. You want to free up as much mental space as reasonable for the important stuff to remember, like feeding yourself and not just baby. Having your annual timeline and scheduled commitments at hand will ease the rescheduling process as you quickly maneuver to an open slot to reassign the incomplete task.

Kendall's Experience

Like most mothers, Kendall tended to overpack her schedule without any breathing room. In fact, packing in as much as she could gave her the false reassurance that she was being the perfect mom doing the most for her pregnancy and unborn baby while still maintaining her household; however, until she dismantled her perfect-household disease, the opposite was what she actually felt: disappointment, guilt, and exasperation for not being able to completely fulfill her overloaded schedule. Now that Kendall allowed herself to be an imperfect mama, she accepted and welcomed Rob's help around the house even when things weren't completed to her standards. But despite Rob's assistance, Kendall's schedule was still overstretched. Instead of routine household obligations, it was now filled with back-to-back tasks to prepare for baby's arrival. Unfortunately, without also including wellness breaks into her schedule, Kendall was still operating with depleted resources and didn't have the means to account for the unforeseen curveballs that sometimes disrupted intended plans. In fact, by the time she accepted reality that her schedule was untenable to weather the unexpected storms that came with a high risk pregnancy, she was inching toward burnout and was placed on bedrest for the last month of her prenatal period.

Being advised to restrict her activities was a real wake-up call for Kendall to do less—much less—and she was amenable to resetting her mindset to embrace her Wellness Tree for both herself and her unborn daughter. Plus, being physically restricted to bedrest gave her the incentive to reallocate her time to her well-being with baby. Hence, she gave herself space to create her annual timeline before scheduling each item into a digital calendar. She dedicated each commitment from her timeline to specified times, all color-coded: yellow for baby and pregnancy demands, green for family and household obligations, and orange for personal requirements. Since Kendall tended to overschedule her days without accounting for all of the mundane responsibilities of daily life, we made sure all of the little things were also included—morning routines, daily breakfast, lunch, and dinner, regular ten- to fifteen-minute breaks, travel time, evening demands, and nighttime rituals. To prepare for her real mom life with baby's impending arrival, she had to also incorporate time for her own wellness and upcoming baby care into the schedule to elucidate a real representation of the limited time actually available to her on any given day. Before fully completing her schedule, she had to finally *abandon her to-do list, dedicating specific times for each task in her calendar instead.*

Alas, trying to schedule every single item into her calendar was proving impossible with only twenty-four hours in a day. To squeeze everything into a day's time meant she had to sacrifice time from elsewhere. Yet, there was nowhere else to squeeze time from. Hence, her remaining options were to prioritize tasks that would otherwise be delayed, choose to delegate specific tasks, or completely remove lower priority tasks altogether. When all of her daily, weekly, and monthly activities and obligations were finally accounted for into her detailed scheduler, Kendall was faced with the fact that she had been undertaking an unwinnable battle against reality. Since she couldn't realistically add more hours to her already full schedule, this realization eased her critical self-judgments of not being and doing enough for her anticipated child. As she prepared for her daughter's arrival, she adopted a more realistic expectation of herself and adjusted the demands on her time. She also felt more supported by Rob now that he was less reliant on her simply because he became more involved with their household obligations. In the end, having dismissed her perfect-household disease while scheduling her motherhood obligations realistically, Kendall was able to fit what she needed into her calendar while preserving her wellness and relationship with her family in the process.

When you schedule a task, you're informing yourself that it will be done at that specified time. It also gives you a dose of reality that there isn't much time in a day to tackle the mountain of tasks from a to-do list. Again, there are only twenty-four hours in a day, 168 hours in a week. Do the math: no wonder the time goes by quickly while you wrongly blame yourself for not being enough. After inserting all of your monthly and weekly commitments from your annual timeline into your daily planner or digital scheduler, you'll see how little time remains for your and baby's daily obligations. Of course, no schedule is set in stone just as no forecast is 100 percent accurate. By acknowledging that seasons evolve throughout the year, you'll have a calmer means of sorting through the scheduling changes from your planned commitments visibly in front of you. All of this might seem like extra work initially, especially when you're a new mom; however, with practice, it will become a natural habit that will support your motherhood sanity while freeing you from intrusive worries and anxiety. Knowing how to keep your motherly apples, branches, and trunk intact comes with experience. Through repetition, the process of scheduling won't be as tedious. It'll just be in your muscle memory.

Rolling with Reality

No plan is ever foolproof because the nature of life is unpredictable, uncertain, and constantly evolving, especially where young children are involved. One moment, you're feeling steady, all seems to be running smoothly, and you might even pat yourself on the shoulder for your impressive planning skills. The very next moment, you're disoriented when your day gets derailed as you try to regain footing after deviating from the schedule. You might be filled with exasperation, disenchantment, and apprehension during these impromptu moments while trying to rigidly stick to the plan. However, while you're stuck with anxious thoughts in a spiraling ruminado, time doesn't stop ticking and keeps flowing moment to moment with or without your presence. As you're swept further and further, your anxiety monster will keep running circles around you with catastrophic delusions of everything that is now wrong.

To prevent anxious, disastrous thoughts from taking over, you have to stay grounded and keep your roots from lifting by unexpected storms. Just as branches from a healthy tree blows with spontaneous gusts of wind, rolling with reality when things don't go as planned is the path of least resistance. You might lose some leaves and apples along your motherhood journey; however, as long as you're flowing with the breeze, you're less likely to run the risk of also losing your trunk. This means embracing reality and adjusting expectations so you can ease your stress and prioritize getting the truly imperative tasks done. When you let go of rigid expectations, you're clearing the way for the sun to shine on new possibilities and solutions that may otherwise be hidden behind dark ominous clouds.

Let's say you're immersed in work with your team to meet a client's deadline tomorrow morning and your phone rings, displaying baby's daycare on the caller ID. You know if you answer, you'll likely be called away to attend to the matter. Yet, without hesitation, you respond anyway and now must drop your work commitment, take a detour from your planned agenda, and pick up your child. You can huff and puff all you want, except no huffing or puffing will change the reality of the situation, and instead, will waste the energy you'll need to perhaps wrap up your work assignment later that evening. A healthier mindset would be to roll with reality, accept the situation for what it is, and adjust your expectations for your evening plans. In fact, whenever we get derailed from our intended schedule, we really only have two choices: modify your expectations or add more hours to the day. Since one isn't rational, then the pragmatic approach is to adjust your expectations.

In truth, all of the tools you've acquired in each chapter have already prepared you to roll with reality. You've learned to embrace uncertainty, adopt flexibility, lean into the moment, challenge unrealistic judgments, shift your mindset, and assert protective boundaries to reclaim wellness on your motherhood journey. Adjusting your expectations to reflect reality when you have to deviate from plans eliminates the space for your anxious monster to trick you with deceptive perspectives. How do you want to spend your time? Beating yourself up with disappointment or saving your energy for rational solutions?

Here's a suggestion: focus on scheduling your obligations *and* your desires. Having only twenty-four hours to each day, you can choose how you intend to spend that time. Playing with baby or replying to work emails? Volunteering in your community or starting a new personal hobby? Attending a birthday party or having a candlelit dinner with your partner? Spiraling with intrusive anxious thoughts or protecting your sanity to authentically bond with baby and family? Although you can't do it all, you can fit what's doable within the limited time that is realistic.

Practice these strategies to adjust your expectations and roll with reality the next time your plans become disrupted. You never know when an unforeseen storm will surprise you. When the unexpected sneaks up on you, choosing to flow with the winds will keep you grounded, whereas remaining rigidly planted will likely pull up your roots and leave you with broken branches:

1. When unexpected demands put your plans on a detour, use your schedule to inform you of the options available to you. You cannot change the reality of the situation; however, you can adapt to plan B or C or D as long as you're flexible to roll with other options. It might not be realistic to reschedule your unmet plan immediately, and if so, choose to delay it or prioritize it and move other scheduled tasks to a later time.

2. If your schedule is completely filled for months, then you have three choices: (1) remove or outsource the task of lower priority or value; (2) delay the task to your next availability in several months; or my favorite, (3) start saying, "No, thank you" to additional requests. This reality requires you to adjust your expectations and evaluate each demand on your time according to your values and priorities. What is worth maximizing? What deserves minimizing? Roll with the reality that not everything can be scheduled immediately.

3. Moving forward, whenever you see your schedule filling up, use this as an alert that there's no more room to add more tasks unless something else is rescheduled to a later time or sacrificed completely. Remember prioritizing your Wellness Tree is also prioritizing your bond with baby. Without your leaves, apples, and branches, you won't have the resources needed to care for baby and family. Adjust any impractical expectations that you have *unlimited* time. Once your limit is reached, it's time to say, "No, thank you" to further requests of lower value and roll with this reality.

Madelyn's Experience

Having embraced her nanny's way of doing things, Madelyn had envisioned a seamless return to her professional career following her six-month maternity leave. Armed with her newly acquired skills and motherhood doctrine, she was carefully planning her schedule to balance work and life with her now seven-month-old baby. Yet, within a month of returning to work, she was overwhelmed once again from having to juggle work responsibilities and mom life demands. She was constantly sleep-deprived, waking up early before baby or staying up late into the nights to finish work assignments. She felt guilty for not being able to devote as much quality time to be with baby in the mornings and evenings. She also felt frustrated by the new workload from her job that took up more than the regular 9–5 hours that she had anticipated. Despite having her annual timeline and scheduling guidelines at hand, Madelyn was stretched thin to a breaking point once again with her anxiety monster lurking closely behind ready to infiltrate her sanity.

While unpacking her updated motherhood load and new professional workload to discern her current obligations, what Madelyn discovered was that her annual timeline and schedule had evolved with vastly changed responsibilities. She had a different set of unpredictable demands unique to a mobile baby who was much more vocally assertive. Her professional work commitments regularly bled into her baby care and sleep hours. To make matters worse, her schedule was not only completely filled for months, she also kept accepting new work assignments to defuse the discrimination against working mothers.

The thing Madelyn wasn't committed to was rolling with reality. Each time an unexpected storm struck, which occurred quite often with a seven-month-old baby, she felt less capable while intrusive anxious worries consumed more of her mind. To restore her Wellness Tree, we revisited her Values Clarification Worksheet to remind her of the goals that were meaningful while modifying those that no longer served her. We also had to consider adjusting her rediscovered identity to reflect her current life goals with baby and career. With this in mind, Madelyn reworked her annual timeline to comprise all of her current motherhood and professional duties.

However, like most mamas, Madelyn had a tough time scheduling all of her obligations into a twenty-four-hour day and had to choose to delay, delegate, or delete specific tasks of less priority. Even with a nanny, she *had to give her schedule more room for breaks and sudden changes to better manage the unexpected storms that were common for this period of motherhood. Although Madelyn's schedule was still packed, she gave herself more breathing room to reclaim the flexibility needed to bend with the winds that naturally came. Having a more practical timeline and schedule, she was also more aware of what to expect during specific periods of the week, month, and year. Accepting that sometimes her commitment would go more toward work while others would be devoted more to baby, she was better equipped to disregard the unwarranted disappointments and guilt trips from her anxiety monster. Instead of feeling like she was constantly spiraling in circles, Madelyn learned to roll with reality, which provided the sanity and bandwidth needed to continue bonding with her precious baby for the long haul.*

Remember your boundary mom doctrine? Time dedicated for your well-being requires time to be sacrificed elsewhere. It's unlikely you'll have everything scheduled and completed immediately and that's a reality we all have to roll with. Keep the timeline and schedule flexible—because life happens. As long as you have an adaptable mindset for the unforeseen storms that arise, you'll be in a better position to stay grounded from intrusive negative judgments while making room for the unexpected. With a comprehensive timeline in hand and a detailed schedule in front of you, you'll be less likely to commit to a plan that isn't truly important. Make it your year-end review to reflect on the year past and the year ahead, which will give you a chance to update your values and responsibilities along your motherhood journey. It's an essential step to ensure your life is filled with the meaningful commitments that serve you, without making room for your anxious monster to rob you.

Conclusion

Practice Makes Habit

My Experience

My own exposures were just as torturous as the ones I prescribe to my patients. I had to visualize and imagine the unbearable possibility of harm befalling my sweet, innocent babies. I had to live with the uncertainty of not knowing what might happen to them one day. I had to accept the reality that they could die before I do. These thoughts would be hard to tolerate for any mama. For those of us with anxious intrusive thoughts, we must repeatedly practice confronting them until the painful thoughts lose their power. That was the only way I reclaimed my wellness from OCD's power so that my motherhood journey could be the bliss I had dreamed of without OCD's torment.

Whenever my OCD monster switched gears and threw me fresh content to fear, I adapted my strategy to confront whatever the newest theme of intrusive thoughts involved. After a while and following much anguish and tears, the dreaded thoughts became softer, more bearable, and much less invasive. Practicing a flexible mindset without having to focus on every detail of my twin sons also organically corrected my urge to seek reassurances in other ways. Simply put, I no longer felt the need to listen to my OCD monster the more I put my own tools to practice. Rather than wasting time on OCD's absurd demands, I chose to be free from them so that I could bond authentically with my sweet babies without OCD's interference. Although facing my worst fears was a daunting task, living a life with agonizing intrusive thoughts was much, much worse. One that interfered with my attachment to my twin boys. Whenever I reflect back on those early days suffering from postpartum OCD, practicing the arduous tasks that flexed my mental muscles had been worth every tear and heartbreak. That's the paradox in the anxious monster's bag of tricks.

Old habits are hard to change, simply because they've been repeatedly practiced and reinforced over time. Habits are familiar, and familiarity breeds comfort and complacency. On the other hand, our brain's neuroplasticity makes it possible to build new habits through time and practice, as you've learned earlier in the book. To facilitate change, simply having insight about what needs to change isn't enough. I'm sure you've heard the advice to eat better, exercise and sleep more, and even take time for self-care; however, just because you know what is needed to be healthier doesn't necessarily mean it'll be implemented. For practical change to take place, we have to practice creating new habits; in this case, habits in thinking and being.

When you first begin this practice, you might not fully grasp how avoidance or escape methods actually reinforce your anxiety monster's power. You might not realize the intrusive thoughts you have are likely thoughts that many mamas have also had—only you notice them more because you've tried to resist them more. You might not notice the mind traps in your thought process that trigger your unpleasantly felt emotions. Likewise, you might not initially feel comfortable leaning into those dreaded emotions to expand your comfort zone and flexibility. Like most mamas, you also might not recognize how deeply impacted you are by the classic supermom ideals causing your perfect-household disease. You might have doubts about being able to rediscover your mom+ identity or implement your boundary mom doctrine. Finally, even with a schedule, you might still have trouble believing that you only have twenty-four hours in a day and try to sneak additional tasks into your daily and weekly plan without sacrificing others.

Yes, the tools and guidelines here might initially feel foreign because they are, and you might find them challenging at first because they're new to you. Though just like any new skill worth having, the more you practice and flex your mental muscles, the more familiar, natural, and proficient you'll become. The goal isn't to achieve perfection because practice does *not* make perfect and striving for perfection is a losing battle that will trigger your deeply embedded insecurities and faulty beliefs. Instead, embrace "practice makes habit."

I acknowledge that practice is hard, tedious, and requires much effort in the beginning. Yet, having your anxious monster constantly lurking around your mind consumes even more energy—physical, mental, and emotional energy that can be devoted to your baby and family. Hence, diverting your energy from the spiral of anxiety to practicing these tools will only provide you with healthier habits that serve you *and* baby. Every step of the way, every mental muscle you flex will help you get closer and closer to the authentic mom life that nurtures your bond with those you love. The more you practice these skills and strategies, the better you'll be at changing the unhelpful habits that maintain those dreaded intrusive thoughts and worries.

As your new and healthier thinking skill strengthens over time, you'll be able to stop the spiral of anxiety with more ease and less effort. To reclaim your authentic mom life from unwarranted worries and intrusive thoughts, keep practicing the strategies that will activate your oxygen mask and replenish your reserves to ensure long-term wellness. Don't wait to reach chronic stress and rage before allocating time for your mental, emotional, and physical well-being. Trust me, once you've reached burnout, the toll it takes on your overall health becomes immeasurable, and the time it takes to heal and recover is even more energy-consuming. In fact, chronic stress and burnout can lead to premature death, and if that's the case, what use are you? Without *you* functioning optimally, how will your family then manage all of the household tasks that you magically handled?

If you're not convinced, think of the last time you felt chronic stress, burnout, and perhaps even compassion fatigue. How effective were you at juggling all the demands of motherhood without a healthy reserve tank?

How did you feel about the multitude of requests coming at you from your child, partner, work, community, or anyone else who feels they have a right to your time? How was your connection with your family? What was your relationship like with yourself? To live a mom life that's meaningful and honors your whole self, you have to reclaim your wellness throughout your motherhood journey starting now.

Remember, you're human and a mom who doesn't need reasons to restore your energy. Plus, imagine the healthy bond a well-rested mama would have with her family. Because if you don't, who would? When you don't prioritize your wellness, you're instead in agreement with the societal bias that neglecting mothers is justifiable. Therefore, align yourself to be celebrated regularly without undue guilt and stress—not just on your birthday or Mother's Day. With more physical, mental, and emotional reserves, you'll uncover more moments of sunshine and rainbows amid the clouds in your authentic mom life with baby. Through consistent practice, you'll cultivate the natural habit of stopping the spiral of anxiety as you reclaim wellness on your motherhood journey.

Epilogue

The Problem with "Self-Care"

Many moms know that taking time for "self-care" is essential to your wellness. By this point, you've read about this notion time and again in the preceding pages. Now that you've arrived at the end of this book, have you started to prioritize time for your well-being? Me time? Have you intentionally scheduled self-care? More crucially, have you actually kept time for yourself despite the urge to spend it on other mom life demands when they regularly pile on? In essence, are you really committed to your care and wellness by utilizing your oxygen mask first before running out of fuel from constantly tending to baby and family's well-being above your own?

If you haven't, why not? Here again, just because you're aware that self-care is vital to your motherhood wellness doesn't necessarily mean you'll implement it regularly. The problem with self-care is that it sounds optional and carries the weight of guilt due to the common perspective that taking time for yourself is selfish and a sheer luxury when you have needy baby and family obligations at hand. Now instead of "self-care," what if you shifted your mindset to "self-maintenance"? Does prioritizing time for self-maintenance to replenish your bandwidth and fuel tank seem more mandatory?

If you're still not convinced, let's take a machine, like a vehicle, into consideration. You turn off your car daily and give it breaks in between driving. You refuel it weekly when the gas tank is empty or recharge it to power it back up. You even schedule regular car maintenance every few months to ensure its safety and dependability. How are you, a mortal human, any different? Do you give yourself the same consideration of regular self-maintenance? If you don't, then you will indeed burn out over time, become inoperable, and possibly even be in disrepair.

Like any machine that breaks down, you will then need to spend time in a repair shop if you wish to be operable, which will be even more time-consuming and costly. In fact, while mechanical parts can be replaced when damaged, there aren't many human parts that can be usefully replaced. Hence, maintaining yourself is even more imperative than maintaining your vehicle, and is not optional. Frankly, self-maintenance is indispensable to your wellness throughout your motherhood journey and is a fundamental responsibility just like car ownership.

All of the strategies and tools you've acquired from this book have cultivated this self-maintenance mindset free from undue guilt or unnecessary judgment. Remember, when you maintain your well-being, you become a nourished mama who's better equipped to nurture your family and others around you. Essentially, embracing self-maintenance protects the mother-child bond that you value and models a powerful example for your loved ones. Whether you're a new or veteran mom, it's a necessary investment and not a luxury if you want to steadfastly stay the course on your motherhood journey. Therefore, practice scheduling your monthly, weekly, and even daily self-maintenance commitments to refuel your resilience and fortify your foundation, and be sure to do it consistently if you don't want to burn out, break down, and become inoperable or in disrepair. Instead of chanting the untenable expectations that maintain your perfect-household disease, let "self-maintenance" be your empowering mantra.

Ultimately, experiencing less unwarranted guilt for valuing your worth to reclaim wellness equals fewer opportunities for the spiral of anxiety. This is how you can authentically greet baby with a warm hello while you bid goodbye to those worrying intrusive thoughts.

Acknowledgments

First and foremost, I must express my most profound gratitude to my family for graciously enduring my absence over the past year, particularly during the myriad days, weeks, and months when I was completely immersed in writing into the wee hours. To my charming twin boys, your inexplicable empathy and understanding of the significance of this book, crafted at the sacrifice of attending your basketball games, accompanying you on school field trips, and sharing weekend playtimes have truly touched my heart. To my loving husband, you are my anchor, source of strength, and cherished life partner. I am immensely appreciative of your unwavering support, enduring patience, and selfless commitment to nurturing our beautiful children, enabling me to bring this book to fruition.

Second, I am indebted to my parents, especially my mother, who raised me to believe "I can" even during moments when I didn't think it. You have taught me to embrace the necessary boundaries of life that foster strength and resilience, all the while embodying compassion for the limits that exist.

Without my mentor, Dr. Barbara Van Noppen, checking on me during those early postpartum days and prompting reflection on possible intrusive OCD thoughts, my struggles would've likely been prolonged. I deeply value your decades-long guidance and support in my career and our kindred friendship that has evolved to what it is today.

I extend my appreciation to everyone who contributed to the creation of this book. In particular, to my friends and colleagues who generously shared their own motherhood experiences and heartaches: your time and insights have meaningfully enriched the content within these pages.

Above all, my heartfelt gratitude goes to my patients and every mother who has entrusted my guidance in their motherhood journey. This book holds the depth it does because of your stories and tears, and I truly hope it serves as validation to your struggles and experiences, both now and into the future.

I dedicate this book to all mothers, new and seasoned, for your tireless labor that ensures the wellness of your children, family, and others, while still firmly staying the course on this rollercoaster journey called motherhood. Now, it's time to reclaim your own wellness.

References

Ali, E. 2018. "Women's Experiences with Postpartum Anxiety Disorders: A Narrative Literature Review." *International Journal of Women's Health* 10: 237–249. https://doi.org/10.2147/IJWH.S158621.

Anokye, R., E. Acheampong, A. Budu-Ainooson, E. I. Obeng, and A. G. Akwasi. 2018. "Prevalence of Postpartum Depression and Interventions Utilized for Its Management." *Annals of General Psychiatry* 17: 18. https://doi.org/10.1186/s12991-018-0188-0.

Aztlan-James, E. A., M. McLemore, and D. Taylor. 2017. "Multiple Unintended Pregnancies in U.S. Women: A Systematic Review." *Women's Health Issues* 27(4): 407–413. https://doi.org/10.1016/j.whi.2017.02.002.

Besen-Cassino, Y., and D. Cassino. 2014. "Division of House Chores and the Curious Case of Cooking: The Effects of Earning Inequality on House Chores Among Dual-Earner Couples." *AG About Gender International Journal of Gender Studies* 3(6): 25–53. https://doi.org/10.15167/2279-5057/ag.2014.3.6.176.

Bianchi, S. M., L. C. Sayer, M. A. Milkie, and J. P. Robinson. 2012. "Housework: Who Did, Does or Will Do It, And How Much Does It Matter?" *Social Forces* 91(1): 55–63. https://doi.org/10.1093/sf/sos120.

Coltrane, S. 2000. "Research on Household Labor: Modeling and Measuring the Social Embeddedness of Routine Family Work." *Journal of Marriage and the Family* 62(4): 1208–1233. https://doi.org/10.1111/j .1741-3737.2000.01208.x.

Declercq, E. R., C. Sakala, M. P. Corry, S. Applebaum, and P. Risher. 2002. *Listening to Mothers: Report of the First National U.S. Survey of Women's Childbearing Experiences.* New York: Maternity Center Association.

Doan, L., and N. Quadlin. 2018. "Partner Characteristics and Perceptions of Responsibility for Housework and Child Care." *Journal of Marriage and Family* 81(1): 145–163. https://doi.org/10.1111/jomf.12526.

Dubber, S., C. Reck, M. Müller, and S. Gawlik. 2015. "Postpartum Bonding: The Role of Perinatal Depression, Anxiety and Maternal-Fetal Bonding During Pregnancy." *Archives of Women's Mental Health* 18(2): 187–195. https://doi.org/10.1007/s00737-014-0445-4.

Dunatchik, A., and S. Speight. 2020. "Re-examining How Partner Co-Presence and Multitasking Affect Parents' Enjoyment of Childcare and Housework." *Sociological Science* 7: 268–290. https://doi.org/10 .15195/v7.a11.

Firoz, T., A. McCaw-Binns, V. Filippi, L. A. Magee, M. L. Costa, J. G. Cecatti, M. Barreix, et al. 2018. "A Framework for Healthcare Interventions to Address Maternal Morbidity." *International Journal of Gynecology and Obstetrics* 141(1): 61–68. https://doi.org/10.1002ijgo .12469.

Işık, M., and Van Education and Research Hospital. 2018. "Postpartum Psychosis." *Eastern Journal of Medicine* 23(1): 60–63. https://doi.org/10 .5505/ejm.2018.62207.

Scheinost, D., R. Sinha, S. N. Cross, S. H. Kwon, G. Sze, R. T. Constable, and L. R. Ment. 2017. "Does Prenatal Stress Alter the Developing Connectome?" *Pediatric Research* 81(1–2): 214–226. https://doi.org/10 .1038/pr.2016.197.

Walker, R., M. Blackie, and M. Nedeljkovic. 2021. "Fathers' Experience of Perinatal Obsessive-Compulsive Symptoms: A Systematic Literature Review." *Clinical Child and Family Psychology Review* 24: 529–541. https://doi.org/10.1007/s10567-021-00348-2.

Jenny Yip, PsyD, ABPP, has fought her own personal battle with obsessive-compulsive disorder (OCD). Inspired by her childhood struggles and motivated to help others, Yip established the Renewed Freedom Center in 2008 and the Little Thinkers Center in 2016 to provide cutting-edge treatments for children, parents, and families. Yip is on the board of directors of the International OCD Foundation (IOCDF), where she facilitates the Perinatal OCD Task Force, and is a clinical fellow of the Anxiety and Depression Association of America (ADAA). A sought-after speaker on mental health, family dynamics, pediatric development, and maternal wellness, she has delivered numerous impactful presentations around the world.

Yip has received several prestigious awards recognizing her invaluable contributions to the field. Renowned as the go-to expert, Yip is a regular guest on television, podcasts, and in print, national radio, drawing on her extensive twenty-plus-years' experience in evidence-based clinical treatments, teaching, and research. In an effort to raise accurate awareness, eliminate mental health stigmas, and provide practical parenting tools, Yip is tirelessly involved in various projects to provide effective strategies for a stressless life. Her most paramount endeavor lies in nurturing her twin boys to live compassionately, empowered by healthy and meaningful boundaries.

Real change *is* possible

For more than forty-five years, New Harbinger has published proven-effective self-help books and pioneering workbooks to help readers of all ages and backgrounds improve mental health and well-being, and achieve lasting personal growth. In addition, our spirituality books offer profound guidance for deepening awareness and cultivating healing, self-discovery, and fulfillment.

Founded by psychologist Matthew McKay and Patrick Fanning, New Harbinger is proud to be an independent, employee-owned company. Our books reflect our core values of integrity, innovation, commitment, sustainability, compassion, and trust. Written by leaders in the field and recommended by therapists worldwide, New Harbinger books are practical, accessible, and provide real tools for real change.

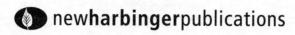 **newharbinger**publications

MORE BOOKS from
NEW HARBINGER PUBLICATIONS

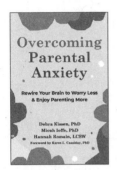
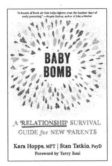
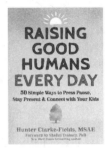
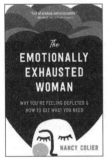
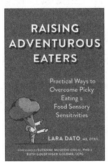
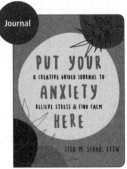